100 CASES
in Radiology

D1387485

100 CASES
in Radiology

Robert Thomas
Specialist Registrar, Guy's and St Thomas' Hospital, London, UK

James Connelly
Specialist Registrar, Guy's and St Thomas' Hospital, London, UK

Christopher Burke
Specialist Registrar, Guy's and St Thomas' Hospital, London, UK

100 Cases Series Editor:
Professor P John Rees MD FRCP
Professor of Medical Education, King's College London School of Medicine at
Guy's, King's and St Thomas' Hospitals, London, UK

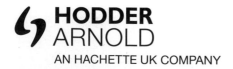
HODDER
ARNOLD
AN HACHETTE UK COMPANY

First published in Great Britain in 2012 by
Hodder Arnold, an imprint of Hodder Education, Hodder and Stoughton Ltd,
a division of Hachette UK
338 Euston Road, London NW1 3BH

http://www.hodderarnold.com

Hachette UK's policy is to use papers that are natural, renewable and recyclable products and made
from wood grown in sustainable forests. The logging and manufacturing processes are expected to
conform to the environmental regulations of the country of origin.

Whilst the advice and information in this book are believed to be true and accurate at the date of
going to press, neither the author[s] nor the publisher can accept any legal responsibility or liability
for any errors or omissions that may be made. In particular, (but without limiting the generality of
the preceding disclaimer) every effort has been made to check drug dosages; however it is still
possible that errors have been missed. Furthermore, dosage schedules are constantly being revised
and new side-effects recognized. For these reasons the reader is strongly urged to consult the
drug companies' printed instructions, and their websites, before administering any of the drugs
recommended in this book.

British Library Cataloguing in Publication Data
A catalogue record for this book is available from the British Library

Library of Congress Cataloging-in-Publication Data
A catalog record for this book is available from the Library of Congress

ISBN-13   978-1-4441-2331-9

1 2 3 4 5 6 7 8 9 10

Commissioning Editor: Joanna Koster
Project Editor: Jenny Wright
Production Controller: Francesca Wardell
Cover Design: Amina Dudhia
Index: Laurence Errington

Typeset in 10/12pt RotisSerif by Phoenix Photosetting, Chatham, Kent
Printed and bound in India by Replika Press

What do you think about this book? Or any other Hodder Arnold title?
Please visit our website: www.hodderarnold.com

CONTENTS

ACKNOWLEDGEMENTS

The authors would like to thank the following people for their help in the preparation of the text and illustrations: Dr Elisa Perry (consultant radiologist at Guys' and St Thomas' Hospital), Dr Russel Houghton (consultant radiologist at Guys' and St Thomas' Hospital), Dr Haran Jogeesvaran (consultant radiologist at Guys' and St Thomas' Hospital), Dr Andrew McGrath (consultant interventional radiologist at Guys' and St Thomas' Hospital), Dr H.K. Mohan (consultant nuclear medicine physician at Guys' and St Thomas' Hospital) and Dr David Howlett (consultant radiologist at Eastbourne Hospital). Many of the images were produced during the authors' time as registrars at Guy's and St Thomas' Hospital. Without the support of the hospital in allowing the use of anonymized images this book would not have been possible.

CASE 1: DETERIORATING SHORTNESS OF BREATH IN A SMOKER

History

You are asked to review a 72-year-old man on the post-take ward round. He was admitted last night with increasing shortness of breath. His breathing has been getting worse for many years now, and he notices that it is especially bad in the winter. His general practitioner (GP) has diagnosed asthma and has been managing him at home. He recalls having several courses of antibiotics over the last few years.

His recent problems started 3 days ago with a cough productive of green sputum. He has felt generally unwell and his breathing has deteriorated significantly. He cannot climb the stairs at home now and slept on the sofa last night. His GP saw him this morning and referred him to hospital as an infective exacerbation of asthma. He continues to smoke despite advice, and has a 50 pack-year history. There is no other relevant past medical history. He takes a salbutamol inhaler when needed but today this was of little help.

Examination

Some blood tests were performed and a chest radiograph was requested (Figure 1.1). His white cell count is 16.3 × 10⁹/L, neutrophil count 89 per cent and haemoglobin 14.2 g/dL.

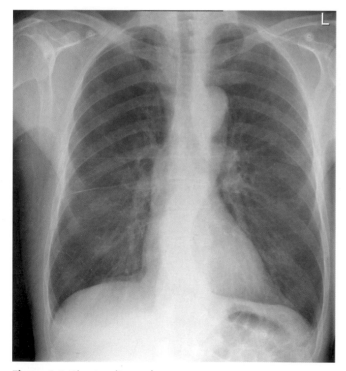

Figure 1.1 Chest radiograph.

Questions

- What does this radiograph show?
- What is the likely diagnosis and how can this be confirmed?

ANSWER 1

This is a posterior–anterior (PA) chest radiograph of an adult male. The lungs are hyper-expanded as evidenced by visualizing more than six anterior ribs above the diaphragm. The distance between the apex of the hemidiaphragm and a line drawn from the costo-phrenic to the cardiophrenic angle is less than 1.5 cm, in keeping with diaphragmatic flattening. The lung parenchyma demonstrates bullous emphysematous disease, most marked in the upper zones. There is no evidence of consolidation, collapse or pneumo-thorax. The cardiomediastinal borders are within normal limits, and both hila are of normal morphology. This chest radiograph suggests a diagnosis of chronic obstructive pulmonary disease (COPD).

COPD is a combination of increased mucus production, small airway obstruction and emphysematous change, with a slow and progressive history of increasing shortness of breath, usually in association with significant tobacco usage. Most commonly, the emphysematous component is 'centrilobular', with irreversible destruction of normal lung most in the apical segments of the upper lobes. On computed tomography (CT) this is clearly seen as central black holes of destroyed lung 'punched-out' from normal paren-chymal architecture (Figure 1.2), although a CT is not a necessary investigation in most cases of COPD. Sometimes the clinical symptoms of COPD are confused with asthma, which usually starts in childhood and shows greater reversibility of airflow obstruction. Some patients develop asthma later in life, and in practice both conditions may coexist or be difficult to differentiate.

The most important investigation in a patient with COPD is lung function test-ing. Spirometry shows the reduced forced expiratory volume in 1 second : forced vital capacity (FEV_1 : FVC) ratio charac-teristic of obstructive conditions. There is an increase in the total lung capacity (TLC) and residual volume (RV) in COPD as a result of air trapping.

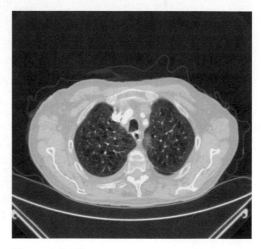

Reversibility to bronchodilators is limited in COPD. Assessment of functional capac-ity is an important part of the evaluation in chronic COPD. In acute exacerbations such as that described, it is important to assess blood gases to look for significant hypoxia and/or carbon dioxide retention.

Figure 1.2 CT scan.

 KEY POINTS

- Flattening of the diaphragms and lung hyperexpansion are characteristic chest radiograph features of COPD.
- COPD is a combination of increased mucus production, small airways obstruction and emphysematous change.
- Lung function tests are the most important investigation in a patient with COPD.

CASE 2: THE BREATHLESS ASTHMATIC

History

A 36-year-old woman presented to the accident and emergency department complaining of progressively increasing breathlessness over the last 2 weeks. This was accompanied by a wheeze and cough productive of white sputum. Her exercise tolerance had reduced and she denied any orthopnoea or chest pain. She had a history of asthma which was usually well controlled with inhalers and had never previously required a hospital attendance. There was no other history of note and she denied ever being a smoker. She lived at home with her husband and two children.

Examination

On examination, her respiratory rate was 22 breaths per minute. She was afebrile and normotensive with a regular pulse rate of 88 per minute. Her cardiovascular and abdominal examinations were normal, but on auscultation of her lungs there was a prolonged expiratory wheeze with reduced air entry at the left base.

A chest radiograph was performed as part of her initial investigations (Figure 2.1).

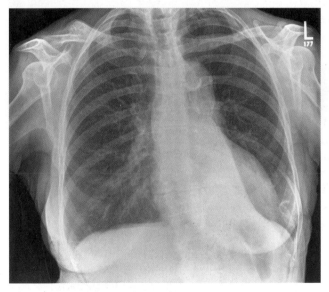

Figure 2.1 PA chest radiograph.

Questions

- What radiological abnormality is present?
- What is the most likely cause considering her history?

ANSWER 2

This patient has left lower lobe collapse. Depending on the airway obstructed, each lobe collapses in a characteristic way. This was originally described by Benjamin Felson, a professor of radiology in the United States in 1973. In the case of the left lower lobe, when there is proximal occlusion, the lobe collapses posteriorly and medially towards the spine. Lying behind the heart, it assumes a triangular shape with a straight lateral border being classically described as a 'sail sign' on posterior–anterior (PA) chest radiograph as shown in Figure 2.2.

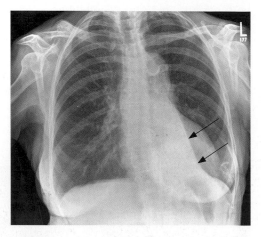

It usually overlies the cardiac shadow and can be easily missed on poorly windowed or under-penetrated films. The collapsed lobe obscures the left medial hemidiaphragm and the horizontal fissure swings downwards with the hilar displaced inferiorly. Other features to help confirm the diagnosis would include mediastinal and tracheal shift towards the side of the collapse, and possible herniation of the contralateral lung across the midline from compensatory hyperinflation. The degree of hilar depression and compensatory hyperaeration is variable depending on the degree of collapse. Less commonly, a stenosing bronchogenic tumour may be seen as a soft tissue density overlying the left hilar point.

Figure 2.2 PA chest radiograph with 'sail sign' indicated.

The causes of lobar collapse are numerous; incidence varies with age and clinical history. Overall, the commonest cause of collapse is related to a proximal stenosing bronchogenic carcinoma, and although the majority of lung cancer is seen in men, the incidence in women is rising. Lung cancer is rarely diagnosed in people younger than 40, but the incidence rises steeply thereafter with most cases (85 per cent) occurring in people over the age of 60 with a past medical history of smoking. In ventilated patients, including neonates, malpositioning of the endotracheal tube can aerate one lung and occlude the contralateral side, while in infants, collapse related to an inhaled foreign body (e.g. a peanut) should always be considered. In older children and young adults, the commonest cause of lobar collapse is as a complication of asthma.

Asthma is a chronic inflammatory disease characterized by reversible airflow limitation and airway hyperresponsiveness. In response to immunological stimuli, mucus hypersecretion from goblet cell hyperplasia can cause airway plugging. Proximal occlusion of a bronchus causes loss of aeration, and as the residual air is gradually absorbed, the lung volume reduces with eventual collapse. Considering the patient's age and clinical history, this is the most likely cause of her left lower lobe collapse.

 KEY POINTS

- Depending on the airway affected, each lobe collapses in a characteristic way.
- The 'sail sign' on a PA chest radiograph is indicative of left lower lobe collapse.
- In paediatric cases, always consider inhaled foreign body as a possible cause of lobar collapse.

History

A 39-year-old woman is sent for an X-ray following a fall. She slipped on some ice while out shopping and raised her right hand to break the fall but her little finger was hyper-flexed in the palm of her hand. She felt an instant sharp and stabbing pain in her little finger, which was centred over the distal and interphalangeal joints. Over the next few hours, her finger began to swell and was increasingly uncomfortable. No other injury was sustained and she attended her local general practitioner (GP) practice for further advice.

Examination

On examination there was soft tissue swelling and a partially flexed little finger that the patient was unable to completely straighten. There was no evidence of skin breach and the patient was otherwise fit and healthy. Concerned that a fracture had been sustained, the GP referred her to hospital for an X-ray and definitive treatment (Figure 3.1a,b).

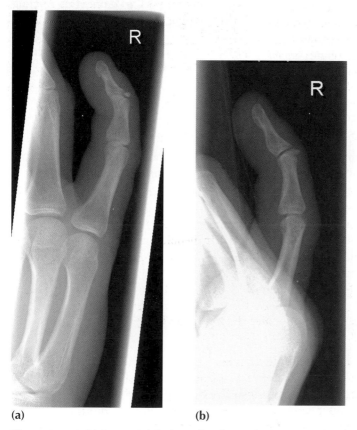

(a) (b)

Figure 3.1 (a) Oblique and (b) lateral radiographs of right little finger.

Questions

- What does this radiograph show?
- What other sites are commonly involved in this form of injury?
- How are X-rays made?

Figure 3.1a is a single oblique radiograph of the right little finger of adequate quality and penetration. There is partial flexion of the distal interphalangeal joint (DIPJ) with a small bony fragment seen in the dorsal aspect of the distal phalynx that is separated from the parent bone. Reduced cortication of the separated surfaces in association with generalized soft tissue swelling is in keeping with an acute fracture, and the bony fragment has been retracted proximally. These appearances are most likely related to a hyperflexion injury, with a fragment of bone avulsed by the extensor tendon at its insertion into the distal phalynx. In summary, there is an avulsion fracture to the distal phalynx of the right little finger.

The term 'avulsion' is used medically to describe one part of the body forcibly detached from another in response to trauma. Commonly seen in the accident and emergency department related to skin degloving from road traffic accidents and nail bed trauma from a crush injury, radiological avulsion fractures occur when a bony fragment is separated from the parent bone in response to forcible contraction of a ligament or tendon. During puberty, secondary ossification centres lay down advancing margins of new bone for continued growth and development, with muscle insertions at this site forming the 'apophysis'. The newly ossified bone is a site of weakness and is vulnerable to separation under extreme force. Any bone subjected to a forceful and usually unbalanced muscle contraction is subject to potential injury, however avulsion fractures are most often seen in active adolescent children commonly at muscle insertions into the pelvis. Sprinters, footballers and tennis players are at greatest risk of such injury. The three commonest sites of pelvis apophyseal avulsion, as shown in Figure 3.2, are:

- ischial tuberosity at the insertion of the adductor magnus muscle of the hamstring;
- anterior inferior iliac iliac spine at the insertion of the rectus femoris muscle; and
- anterior superior iliac spine at the sartorius muscle insertion.

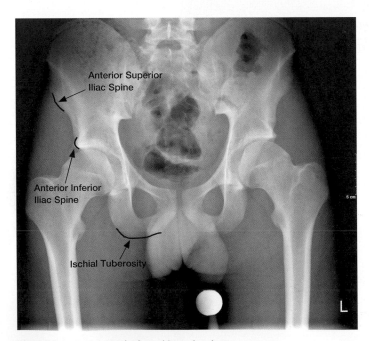

Figure 3.2 Annotated plain film of pelvis.

First discovered by the German physicist W.C. Roentgen in 1895, the discovery of X-rays changed the landscape of medicine forever. To train as a radiologist, the basic physics of X-ray production need to be understood. Every atom is made up of a positively charged nucleus with numerous negatively charged electrons of different energy levels electro-statically held in place around it. Superheating a metal filament (e.g. tungsten) allows a negatively charged electron to free itself from the atom, and this can be accelerated along an X-ray tube attracted by a positively charged 'anode' target plate (also commonly made of tungsten). The fast-moving electron strikes the target plate with such force that it can eject a static electron from a target plate atom out of its normal stable trajectory around its nucleus. This makes the target atom unstable, and to protect itself, another static electron encircling the same nucleus will demote itself from a higher energy band to plug the hole left by the ejected electron. In doing so, it releases energy in the form of a single photon called an 'X-ray'.

Rapidly repeating this procedure can generate an X-ray beam, which when passed through a human body can generate an image on X-ray sensitive material, as the X-rays interact with tissues of differing densities (e.g. bone versus fat).

 KEY POINTS

- Avulsion describes the forcible detachment of one part of the body from another in response to trauma.
- A high index of suspicion of a pelvic apophyseal avulsion in athletic but skeletally immature adolescents is advisable.
- X-Rays were discovered in 1895 by W.C. Roentgen.

History

A 75-year-old man presents complaining of difficulty swallowing together with intermittent regurgitation of undigested food, often some time after eating. This has been slowly worsening. There is occasionally choking and coughing at night. There is no associated pain or heart burn and no history of weight loss or chest symptoms. He has a 30 pack-year smoking history.

Examination

He looks well. The neck and chest examination is normal. No oropharyngeal abnormality is seen on visual examination. The abdomen is soft and non-tender.

A recent chest X-ray is unremarkable. You organize a contrast swallow test (Figure 4.1).

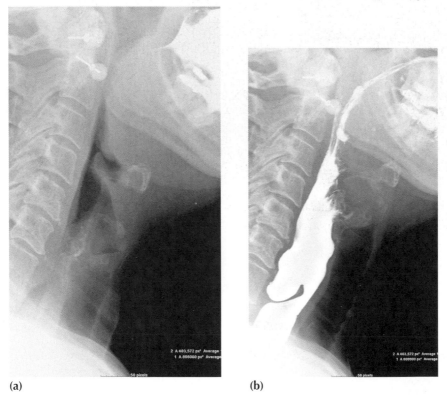

(a)   (b)

Figure 4.1 (a–c) Three sequential lateral projections and (d) an anterior–posterior (AP) projection contrast swallow images. (*continued overleaf*)

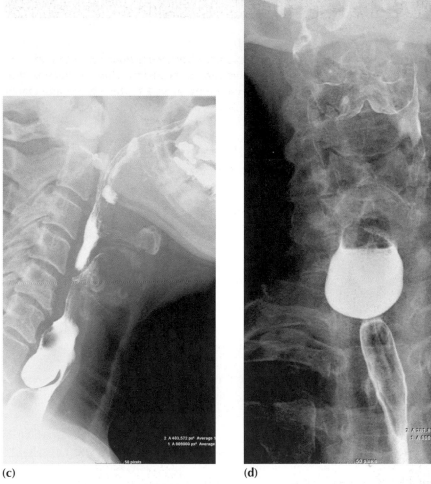

(c)   **(d)**

Figure 4.1 (a–c) Three sequential lateral projections and (d) an anterior–posterior (AP) projection contrast swallow images.

Questions
- What differential diagnosis should be considered?
- What do the images demonstrate?
- What other investigations can be used and what are their relative benefits?

The differential diagnosis for dysphagia is usefully split up into anatomical regions corresponding with the phases of swallowing (i.e. oral, pharyngeal and oesophageal). The type of symptom and the most appropriate investigations depend on whether the problem is primarily oropharyngeal or oesophageal.

Oropharyngeal dysphagia can be caused by:

- central neurological disorders such as stroke, brainstem tumours or degenerative diseases (e.g. Parkinson's disease, multiple sclerosis and Huntington's disease);
- peripheral neurological disorders including peripheral neuropathy, poliomyelitis and syphilis;
- systemic disorders such as myasthenia gravis, polymyositis, dermatomyositis or muscular dystrophy;
- oropharyngeal lesions including cricopharyngeal achalasia, tumours, inflammatory masses, Zenker's diverticulum, oesophageal webs, extrinsic structural lesions, anterior mediastinal masses and cervical spondylosis; see Case 66.

Oesophageal dysphagia can be caused by:

- achalasia;
- spastic motor disorders, such as diffuse oesophageal spasm, hypertensive lower oesophageal sphincter and nutcracker oesophagus;
- scleroderma;
- obstructive lesions, such as tumours, strictures, lower oesophageal rings (Schatzki rings), oesophageal webs, foreign bodies, vascular compression and mediastinal masses.

Endoscopy is the investigation of choice for both oropharyngeal dysphagia, which is typically investigated in the ear, nose and throat department, and oesophageal dysphagia, which is investigated in the upper GI gastroenterology department. If endoscopy does not provide the answer, or the patient refuses the test, then a contrast swallow test can be done to visualize swallowing function. Videofluoroscopy is a low X-ray dose film of the very fast swallowing action in the oropharynx and is useful if there is a motor problem or unsafe swallow. A barium swallow is a series of images taken of the oesophagus while swallowing barium contrast.

This patient's symptoms are suggestive of a pharyngeal or oesophageal problem. On the fluoroscopy images there is barium pooling in an oesophageal diverticulum arising from the posterior midline of the upper oesophagus, the typical position for a pharyngeal pouch (Zenker's diverticulum). This is thought to be caused by spasm or uncoordinated peristalsis of the upper oesophageal sphincter and is located in Killian's triangle, formed by the overlap of the oblique muscles of the inferior constrictor muscle and the transverse muscle fibres of the cricopharyngeus muscle.

The patient's symptoms probably reflect progressive increase in size and compressive effect of the pouch. There is also increased risk of aspiration. The treatment is usually surgical excision or endoscopic stapling. The cricopharyngeal muscle may be separated to prevent recurrence. Complications of pouches include aspiration and, rarely, a carcinoma within the pouch.

Diverticula in other positions are possible. A Killian–Jamieson diverticulum is a lateral cervical oesophageal diverticulum just a little lower in position. Pulsion diverticula associated with abnormal oesophageal contractions sometimes form in the lower third of the oesophagus. Pseudodiverticula are rare dilated glandular pouches in the mucosa of the mid oesophagus associated with reflux.

 KEY POINTS

- Although endoscopy is the investigation of choice, contrast swallow tests provide evidence of functional problems that may not be seen on endoscopy and often underlie dysphagia.
- Common symptoms of a pouch are dysphagia, regurgitation and cough.

History

An 81-year-old woman is bought into the accident and emergency department by ambulance from a local nursing home. As a long-term resident of the home she is an active participant in daily activities, and is usually self-caring and independent. Yesterday evening, she sustained a witnessed mechanical fall, tripping over the walking stick of another resident. Despite a small graze to the right side of the head, there was no loss of consciousness and the patient reassured care home staff that she was fine. An incident report was filed. During the night the patient took paracetamol for pain control of a headache but no further action was taken.

In the morning, she complained of continued headache and the care staff noted a general listlessness and drowsiness. During the course of the day this progressed, and the patient was found slumped in her chair before lunch, rousable only to strong verbal commands. Staff were worried and called an ambulance.

Examination

On inspection the patient had a superficial graze to the right side of her forehead. Her Glasgow Coma Scale (GCS) was 11 (motor 5, eyes 3, speech 3). She was apyrexial, pulse 76 regular, normotensive with a normal cardiovascular examination. There was no focal neurological deficit, and both pupils were equal and reactive. An unenhanced computed tomography (CT) scan was performed (Figure 5.1).

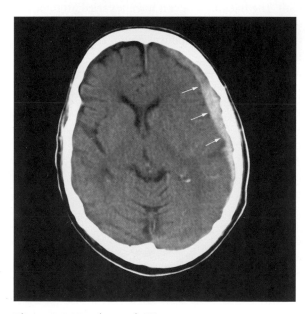

Figure 5.1 Unenhanced CT scan.

Questions

- What does the CT scan demonstrate?
- What is the diagnosis and treatment?

ANSWER 5

This is a single unenhanced image from a cranial CT scan at the level of the basal ganglia. There is an area of asymmetry between the inner table of the skull and the brain in the left cerebral hemisphere. This is more dense than adjacent brain parenchyma but not as dense as the calcified bones of the skull. It conforms to the skull in a concave shape and is predominantly homogeneous in appearance. The adjacent sulci are effaced, as they are not traceable to the brain surface compared to the contralateral side. There is also slight effacement of the left lateral ventricle with some mild midline shift to the right. The brain parenchyma demonstrates preserved grey/white matter differentiation, and there is some generalized cerebral atrophy, demonstrated by increased sulcal spaces seen in the normal right cerebral hemisphere. These findings are in keeping with a subdural haemorrhage with mass effect.

Subdural haemorrhage is defined as a collection of blood in the space between pia mater and dura mater of the leptomeninges.

Laceration of the veins between the two inner layers of the meninges causes blood to accumulate in the subdural space. Although there is an association with direct head trauma and penetrating injury, subdural haematomas are most commonly seen within the elderly population. The brain atrophies with age and becomes more mobile within the skull. The bridging cortical veins are stretched, increasing the risk of both spontaneous rupture and disruption after trivial head injury. Blood is free to track along the surface of the brain within the subdural space and is limited only by the falx and tentorium cerebellum. Cranial CT demonstrates a concave haematoma that, unlike an extradural haemorrhage, crosses suture lines within the skull. The haematoma can have a varied attenuation pattern depending on whether it is an acute, subacute or chronic subdural haemorrhage. For example, Figure 5.2 demonstrates bilateral chronic subdural haemorrhages. In some cases where there is rebleeding, layering of old and fresh blood can be seen, demonstrating an acute-on-chronic picture.

These types of intracranial bleeds tend to be venous in aetiology and blood accumulates slowly in the subdural space. Treatment depends on the neurological deficit caused by the haemorrhage. Patients commonly present with headache, sleepiness and personality change, but if the bleed is large, the conscious level can fluctuate. Signs and symptoms of raised intracranial pressure can occur late and should alert clinicians to the need of urgent evacuation and decompression via a burr hole in a specialist neurosurgical centre. Patients can make a full recovery.

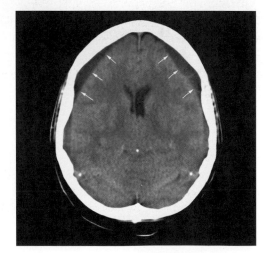

Figure 5.2 CT scan showing bilateral chronic subdural haemorrhages.

🔑 **KEY POINTS**

- In a subdural haemorrhage, blood collects between the pia and dura mater.
- Subdural haemorrhages are more common in the elderly population due to cerebral atrophy.
- Computed tomography demonstrates a concave haematoma unlimited by cranial sutures.

CASE 6: RIGHT UPPER ABDOMINAL PAIN

History

A 45-year-old woman presents to the accident and emergency department complaining of continuous right upper quadrant pain. This has been worsening over the last 12 hours. Previously the patient has had intermittent pain in the same area lasting up to a few hours after eating. She had tried some antacids with no benefit. There has been no vomiting. She complains of irregular bowel pattern, predominantly loose, smelly and rather pallid stool for some months. There is no significant past history and she does not take regular medication.

Examination

The woman appears well but in discomfort with normal observations. The cardiovascular and respiratory examination is normal. The abdomen is soft but focally tender over the right liver edge. The liver is not enlarged. There is no renal angle tenderness.

You arrange tests including an ultrasound of the abdomen (Figure 6.1).

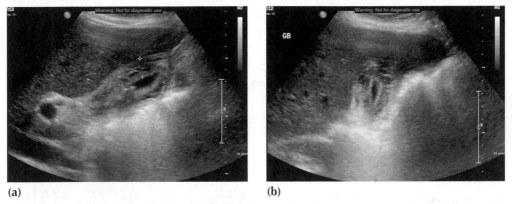

(a) **(b)**

Figure 6.1 Ultrasound views of the liver and gallbladder in longitudinal (a) and transverse (b) planes.

Questions

- What differential diagnoses are you considering?
- What does the ultrasound show?
- Is ultrasound the best investigation to start with?

ANSWER 6

The stool appearance and Murphy's point tenderness point to gallbladder inflammation although the differential includes liver pathology, pancreatitis, gastric or duodenal ulcer, renal obstruction or infection.

The ultrasound shows a partially filled gallbladder with a thickened irregular layered oedematous wall (>3 mm). The gallbladder contains two small stones that reflect virtually all of the beam, giving a shadow appearance behind the stone. A stone is seen in the gallbladder neck and part of the ultrasound examination is to roll the patient onto the right side to see if the stones are mobile. In this case the stone is fixed at the gallbladder neck. These are the appearances of acute obstructive cholecystitis.

For suspected gallbladder or biliary abnormalities, an ultrasound is a good starting investigation. Ultrasound has a very high sensitivity for gallstones whereas at least 20 per cent of gallstones are not seen on computed tomography (CT). Biliary dilatation is also easily seen on ultrasound, appearing as an extra tube running alongside the intrahepatic portal veins (double-barrel sign) or as an extrahepatic dilated common bile duct. Sometimes the cause of obstruction is seen, although the proximity of gas in the stomach, duodenum and hepatic flexure of the colon can often obscure extrahepatic causes. An abdominal radiograph is often included in the work up and is helpful to look for other causes such as renal stones causing colic. Only 30 per cent of gallstones contain enough calcium to be radio-opaque and visible on the abdominal radiograph.

The signs of cholecystitis are also seen frequently on CT that may be done if there is uncertainty as to the diagnosis (Figure 6.2).

Cholecystitis results from obstruction of the cystic duct and in about 90 per cent of cases this is caused by a calculus. In 80 per cent these are cholesterol based, 20 per cent are pigment based. A few cases are caused by sludge that is a fine calcified sediment that forms if the bile becomes very concentrated. The remainder are acalculous cholecystitis, which has all the inflammatory signs without stones and tends to occur in systemic illness, biliary stasis and local or systemic ischaemia. Rarely, gas within the gallbladder or biliary tree is seen if there is added infection.

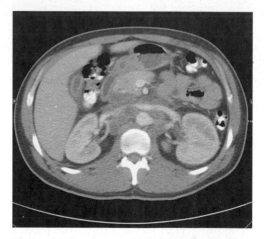

Figure 6.2 Axial contrast CT scan through the gallbladder showing fluid around the gallbladder.

🔑 | **KEY POINTS**

- Ultrasound is a good test for gallbladder and biliary problems.
- Murphy's sign – focal tenderness over the gallbladder – is frequently elicited by the pressure of the ultrasound probe.
- Look on the ultrasound for gallstones, gallbladder wall thickening and oedema as signs of cholecystitis and gas as a sign of infection.

History

A 67-year-old man presents to his general practitioner (GP) with a cough. The man was well known to the doctor as he had been a regular attendee over the course of the previous 12 months with recurrent chest infections. His background included longstanding symptoms of heartburn, dyspepsia and epigastric pain, for which he was prescribed a regular proton pump inhibitor (with some relief). He took no other medications, however, and lived at home with his wife.

Examination

No abnormalities were found on examination of the chest. His respiratory rate was 18 breaths per min with equal and good air entry bilaterally, vesicular breath sounds with no added sounds. He was referred for a chest radiograph (Figure 7.1) but on the basis of the radiograph the reporting radiologist suggested an upper gastrointestinal (GI) contrast swallow examination (Figure 7.2). One day following the barium swallow examination the patient presented acutely in the accident and emergency department with symptoms of epigastric pain, and a computed tomography (CT) scan was performed (Figure 7.3).

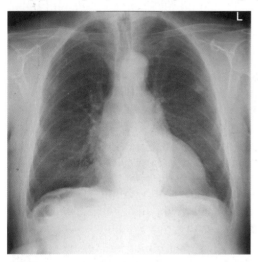

Figure 7.1 Chest radiograph.

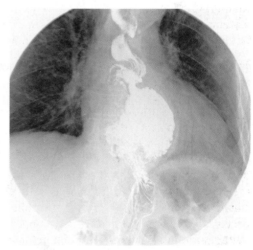

Figure 7.2 Upper GI contrast swallow exam.

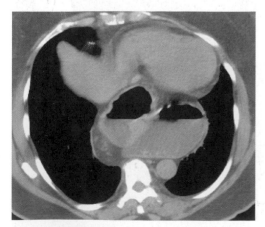

Figure 7.3 CT scan.

Questions

- What does the plain chest radiograph demonstrate (Figure 7.1)?
- Why would the radiologist suggest a barium swallow examination?
- What do the barium swallow spot image (Figure 7.2) and axial enhanced CT image (Figure 7.3) show?

Spot images taken from a barium swallow examination confirm the presence of a sliding hiatus hernia (Figure 7.2). The axial enhanced CT image (Figure 7.3) again demonstrates a large sliding hiatus hernia extending into the thorax. The chest radiograph shows a gas-filled viscus behind the heart shadow consistent with a hiatus hernia. An upper GI contrast examination would confirm the presence of a hiatus hernia and any associated gastro-oesophageal reflux to account for the patient's symptoms.

A hiatus hernia occurs when part of the stomach protrudes into the thoracic cavity through the oesophageal hiatus of the diaphragm. Hiatus hernias are classified either as sliding hernias (where the gastro-oesophageal junction moves above the diaphragm together with part of the stomach) or para-oesophageal or 'rolling' hiatus hernias (where part of the stomach herniates through the oesophageal hiatus and lies beside the oesophagus without movement of the gastro-oesophageal junction). Approximately 95 per cent of hiatus hernias are sliding and the remaining 5 per cent are para-oesophageal.

Plain chest radiographs (as in Figure 7.1) may demonstrate a retro-cardiac mass with or without an air–fluid level. When air is seen within the hernia, the stomach air bubble found below the diaphragm tends to be absent. The hernia is usually positioned to the left of the spine, however larger hernias (particularly when incarcerated) may extend beyond the cardiac confines and even mimic cardiomegaly.

An upper GI barium series (as in Figure 7.2) is the preferred examination in the investigation of hiatus hernia and its sequelae. A single-contrast barium swallow performed with the patient prone is more likely to demonstrate a sliding hiatal hernia than an upright double-contrast examination. The hernia can usually be recognized by the demonstration of mucosal gastric folds. CT scans are useful when more precise cross-sectional anatomic localization is desired.

Most hiatus hernias are actually found incidentally, often being discovered on routine chest radiographs or CT scans performed for unrelated symptoms. When symptomatic, common symptoms include heartburn, dyspepsia or epigastric pain. On occasions, as in this case, the patient may present with recurrent chest infections resulting from aspiration of gastric contents. One sequel of hiatus hernia (particularly the sliding form) is the development of Barrett's oesophagus, which may present with reflux symptoms or dysphagia.

With a para-oesophageal or rolling hernia, part of the stomach rolls into the thorax often anterior to the esophagus and is frequently irreducible. Therefore this type of hernia is more likely to present acutely because of a volvulus or strangulation. A para-oesophageal hiatal hernia is diagnosed by the position of the gastro-oesophageal junction. The cardia of the stomach and gastro-oesophageal junction usually remain in the normal position below the diaphragmatic hiatus and only the stomach herniates into the thorax adjacent to the normally placed gastro-oesophageal junction. This type of hernia, (unlike the sliding form) is not associated with gastro-oesophageal reflux.

 KEY POINTS

- Hiatus hernias are frequently diagnosed incidentally on routine chest radiographs.
- The hernia may be seen as a retro-cardiac mass with or without an air–fluid level.
- An upper GI barium series or barium swallow study is the examination of choice for demonstrating a hiatus hernia, gastro-oesophageal reflux and any associated complications (e.g. Barrett's oesophagus).
- A para-oesophageal or, rarely, sliding hiatal hernia may present acutely because of a volvulus or strangulation.

History

A 59-year-old woman has recently been admitted to the intensive care department. She has chronic renal failure and relies on peritoneal dialysis every night. This morning, while attending her clinic appointment, she complained of a sudden onset of headache and collapsed to the ground, shaking violently. The emergency 'crash' team were called immediately and found the patient unresponsive with generalized jerking movements. The senior doctor decided that she should be paralysed, intubated and ventilated for protective measure, and she was then transferred to the intensive care department for further management. The patient was satisfactorily stabilized, and a central line was placed in her right internal jugular vein for the infusion of intravenous medication and to monitor her central venous pressures. A chest radiograph has been performed to confirm correct placement before its use (Figure 8.1), which you have been asked to report.

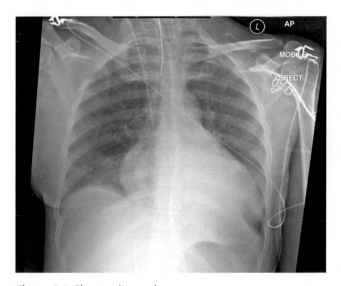

Figure 8.1 Chest radiograph.

Questions

- What additional lines and tubes does this radiograph demonstrate?
- Are the lines and tubes correctly positioned?
- What other common medical equipment may be seen on a radiograph?

Any radiograph can be complicated by additional shadows from foreign lines or drains. Their presence implies that the patient is unwell, and it is important to not only recognize the type of line and common complications associated with its insertion, but its presence on the film should not be a distraction to reporting pathological change (for example, left lower lobe collapse in Figure 8.2). These types of films are often mobile examinations from intensive care (ITU) patients and can be complicated by rotation, poor inspiratory effort and an anterior–posterior (AP) projection. The commonest lines are discussed below, with chest drains discussed in a separate case; see Case 27.

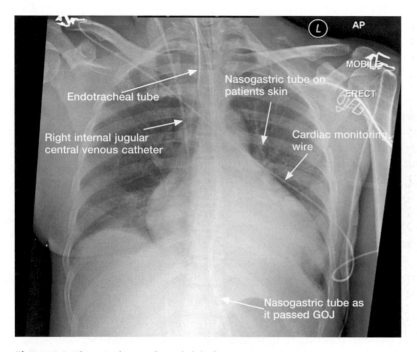

Figure 8.2 Chest radiograph with labels.

- **Endotracheal (ET) tubes:** A patient is intubated for reasons of mechanical ventilation and airway protection usually because they are critically ill or undergoing anaesthesia. Correct placement is critical and an ET tube is recognized on a chest radiograph as a linear opacity projected over the trachea in the midline. Insertion of an ET tube is beyond the scope of this book, but once in the trachea a radiolucent balloon cuff is inflated to maintain stability and a mechanical seal. The tubes are positioned blindly by an airway expert and a chest radiograph is used to confirm its position. Ideally, the tip of an ET tube should be located within the trachea, approximately 1–2 vertebral body heights above the carina. This allows ventilation of both lungs and incorrect placement should be highlighted urgently to the referring clinician. The commonest abnormality is advancement of the ET tube into the right main bronchus preferentially ventilating the right lung only. If not corrected, the patient may be compromised by left lung collapse. An example of an ET tube in the right main bronchus is given in Figure 8.3.

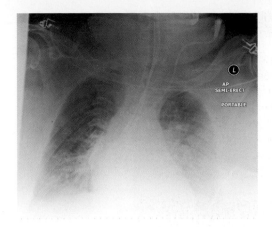

Figure 8.3 Chest radiograph showing ET tube in right main bronchus.

- **Nasogastric (NG) tubes:** These are placed in patients for numerous reasons, most commonly nutritional. Correlating the position of an NG tube does not necessarily require a chest radiograph. Testing the pH of the aspirate can confirm placement within the stomach, thereby avoiding unnecessary radiation exposure. If this is not possible, a chest radiograph should demonstrate the NG tube as a midline linear opacity extending below the left hemidiaphragm. This confirms its presence in the stomach and not in a main stem bronchus, avoiding the catastrophic infusion of nutritional support into the lungs. The tip of an NG tube is not always seen on the chest radiograph, but should lie within the stomach. It can sometimes migrate into the duodenum with gastric peristalsis and should be partially withdrawn.
- **Central lines:** Primarily placed in patients for the infusion of intravenous medication, central lines can also avoid the need for peripheral cannulation and risks of thrombophlebitis. A chest radiograph is performed post insertion to confirm tip position and exclude the most serious complication of pneumothorax. A central line is a radio-opaque density projected paramedially over the internal jugular or subclavian vessels, and can have a wide variety of appearances depending on the side it is inserted and how many lumens the line contains (Figure 8.4). It may also be tunnelled under the skin in the case of a Hickman line, with the possible addition of a buried metallic port (portacath). Recognizing the type of line is important but not essential. Correct tip positioning is critical for optimal infusion. The tip of a central line should ideally lie at the confluence of the inferior and superior vena cava as blood drains into the right atrium. This is identified on a chest radiograph at a point approximately one vertebral body height below the carina. A short line position carries thrombotic risks, while overenthusiastic advancement into the right atrium can encourage myocardial excitation and atrial ectopics.
- **Others:** ET tubes are not suitable for patients requiring long-term ventilatory support and often a tracheotomy is inserted just inferior to the cricoid cartilage. Lying in the midline within the superior mediastinum, a tracheotomy tube appears as a radio-opaque curvilinear density with a buttressed cuff at the skin surface. Its tip should lie within the trachea above the carina.

Figure 8.4 also shows cardiac monitoring and pacing equipment. The two paddle-shaped radio-densities are adhesive conducting pads, and are used to monitor a patient's heart rhythm, control the heart rate through electrical pacing and can be used to deliver an electrical cardioversion shock if necessary. They are correctly positioned here along the electrophysiological axis of the heart. Continuous cardiac monitoring is performed by

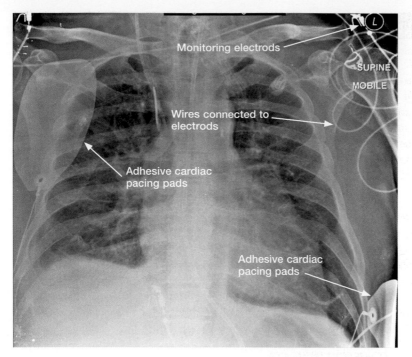

Monitoring electrods

SUPINE

MOBILE

Wires connected to electrods

Adhesive cardiac pacing pads

Adhesive cardiac pacing pads

Figure 8.4 Chest radiograph showing central line.

strategically placed metallic electrodes connected by wires to an external monitoring box. The electrodes can have a variety of appearances and the wires are draped over the patient, often lying erratically over the film. They are seen in Figure 8.4 overlying both humeral heads, and in the right upper quadrant of the abdomen.

KEY POINTS

- The presence of lines indicates an unwell patient.
- It is important not to let lines on a radiograph be a visual distraction to the underlying pathology.
- An ability to recognize all lines and the common complications associated with them is necessary.

CASE 9: WEAKNESS AND SLURRING WHILE OUT FOR A DRINK

History

A 67-year-old man is bought into the accident and emergency department by ambulance with new left-sided limb weakness and a left facial droop. This started 40 minutes earlier while the patient was having a pint in his local pub. Complaining of dizziness for a short while, the patient suddenly fell from his bar stool. The concerned bar tender managed to help him to an armchair and noticed that he was slurring his words and could not use his left arm to help himself up. An ambulance was called, and during this time the patient developed a left-sided facial droop. He remained alert throughout but appeared anxious and disorientated.

The patient is known to the hospital, and has attended previously with attacks of angina. There is no history of myocardial infarction, but he is on tablets for hypertension and dyslipidaemia. He is a smoker and lives at home with his wife. There have been no recent intercurrent illnesses.

Examination

A computed tomography (CT) scan was performed as part of his medical assessment (Figure 9.1).

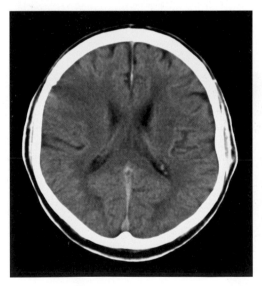

Figure 9.1 CT scan.

Questions
- What does the CT scan show?
- What is a stroke?
- What are the treatment options?

This (Figure 9.1) is a single image from an unenhanced CT scan acquired at the level of the corona radiata. There is a background of generalized involutional change in keeping with the patient's age, and some hemispheric white matter low attenuation suggestive of small vessel disease. Within the right fontal lobe there is a wedge-shaped area of low attenuation with loss of the normal grey/white matter differentiation and extension to the cortical surface. There is mass effect with the adjacent sulci effaced, but no evidence of midline shift or hydrocephalus. There is no evidence of haemorrhage or mass lesion. The image findings are consistent with an acute right middle cerebral artery (MCA) infarction on a background of generalized ischaemic change.

Any vascular interruption within the brain starves distal tissues of blood causing cell death and neurological deficit. This is termed a 'stroke' and is usually thromboembolic (90 per cent) in aetiology,[1] and less commonly haemorrhagic. In the acute setting, unenhanced cranial CT is used to differentiate between the two. Treatment pathways for infarction require antiplatelet therapy, but haemorrhage needs to be excluded to avoid the catastrophic effects of anticoagulation.

Figure 9.2 demonstrates an acute intracerebral haemorrhage within the left cerebral hemisphere. Cranial CT has a high sensitivity (89 per cent) for haemorrhagic stroke. Acute blood within the brain parenchyma appears white on CT (attenuation Hounsfield unit (HU) of 60–70) and stands out against the adjacent darker brain tissue. Treatment for haemorrhagic stroke is usually conservative and supportive.

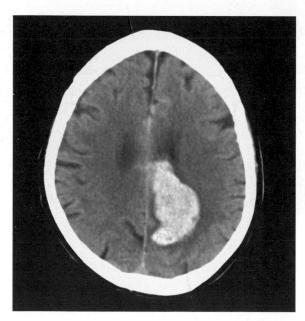

Figure 9.2 CT scan showing acute intracerebral haemorrhage.

In acute infarctive stroke, cranial CT is relatively insensitive (45 per cent at ictus rising to 74 per cent by day 11)[1] and radiological features can vary. A normal cranial CT does not exclude thromboembolic stroke, and should neurological deficit fully resolve within 24 hours, this is termed a transient ischaemic attack (TIA). The significance of patients presenting with a TIA should not be underestimated, and these patients should be considered as an acute medical emergency requiring risk stratification to prevent further nonfatal disabling stroke. In the setting of an acute infarctive stroke or TIA, the cranial CT may be normal. Large thromboembolic strokes classically demonstrate a wedge-shaped area of low density with blurring of the grey/white matter junction. In the image from the CT scan taken from our patient (Figure 9.1), there is loss of grey/white matter differentiation within the right fronto-parietal region compared to the contralateral side. This area is shaded grey in Figure 9.3, which shows the subtle features of an acute thomboembolic stroke.

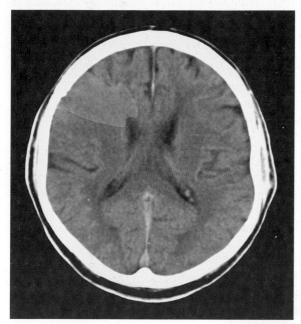

Figure 9.3 CT scan.

In larger infarctive strokes, associated vasogenic oedema can press upon adjacent brain tissue and cause mass effect. The CT findings can usually localize the cerebral artery involved, most commonly the middle cerebral artery (MCA). Figure 9.4 shows an unenhanced axial CT slice demonstrating a well-demarcated area of low attenuation, with loss of the grey/white matter interface and mass effect, in keeping with a large acute left MCA infarct.

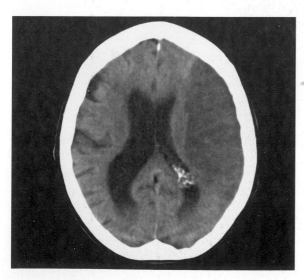

Figure 9.4 Unenhanced axial CT slice.

Many hospitals are now offering thrombolysis therapy for acute thromboembolic stroke. Any history of intracranial haemorrhage is an absolute contraindication, and performing and interpreting a cranial CT is therefore essential prior to treatment. Some other contraindications are listed in Table 9.1 in the criteria taken from the National Institute of Health and Clinical Evidence (NICE) guidance.[2] Thrombolysis therapy has to be administered within 3 hours of symptom onset and speed of brain imaging is very important. Without revascularization, neuronal demyelination causes atrophy of brain tissue with time, and the patient is left with a permanent neurological deficit. In the case of our 67-year-old patient, he may qualify for stroke thrombolysis and a senior stroke physician should initiate this quickly all criteria having been met.

Table 9.1 Criteria taken from the National Institute of Health and Clinical Evidence (NICE) guidance[2]

Inclusion criteria	• Clinical signs and symptoms of a definite acute stroke
	• Clear time of onset
	• Presentation with 3 hours of onset
	• Haemorrhage excluded by CT scan
	• Aged between 18 and 80 years
Contraindications	• Any significant bleeding disorder within the last 6 months
	• Any significant head injury within the last 3 months
	• Current warfarin treatment and an international normalized ratio (INR) >1.4
	• Suspected subarachnoid haemorrhage with a normal CT
	• Acute pancreatitis
	• Bacterial pericarditis or endocarditis
	• Active hepatitis or portal hypertension
	• Documented bleed from abdominal aortic aneurysm (AAA) in last 3 months

 KEY POINTS

- Acute thromboembolic stokes classically demonstrate a wedge-shaped area of low attenuation with blurring of the grey/white matter junction.
- Transient ischaemic attacks (TIAs) should be treated as a medical emergency as a sign of impending stroke.
- Many hospitals now provide systemic thrombolysis for the treatment of acute thromboembolic stroke.

References

1. Dahnert, W. (2007) *Radiology Review Manual*, 6th edn. Philadelphia: Lippincott Williams and Wilkins.
2. National Institute for Health and Clinical Excellence (2007) Alteplase for the treatment of acute ischaemic stroke. www.guidance.nice.org.uk/TA122.

History

A 23-year-old caucasian man presented to the accident and emergency department (A&E) with back pain. Usually fit and healthy, he has suffered from achy throbbing back pain for the last 6 months. Always in the same position in his lower back, it is there intermittently but has increased in frequency over the last 2 weeks. The pain is worse at night and it often wakes him from sleep. He denies any trauma, weight loss or symptoms related to his bladder or bowel movements.

His general practitioner diagnosed occupation-related back pain in relation to the patient's job as a farmer, and recommended rest while prescribing several combinations of analgesia with little symptomatic relief. He does describe marked improvement in his symptoms with aspirin, but the pain often returns after only an hour. Waking up tonight, he was frustrated with the pain at home and attended A&E.

Examination

On examination he looks healthy but in mild discomfort. He has full range of movement with no evidence of bony tenderness on palpation. Cardiovascular, respiratory and abdominal systems are normal. X-ray is shown in Figure 10.1.

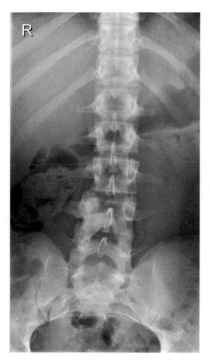

Figure 10.1 Plain radiograph.

Questions

- What does the plain radiograph demonstrate?
- What is your differential for these findings?
- What further investigations need to be performed?

Figure 10.1 is a plain anterior–posterior (AP) radiograph of the lower thoracic and lumbar spine in an adult male patient. The vertebral bodies demonstrate normal alignment in the AP view with normal vertebral body height preserved throughout. There is an abnormality centred on the right L4 pedicle with expansion of the cortex and dense sclerosis. The adjacent transverse process also appears expanded compared to the contralateral side but there is no evidence of periosteal reaction. The psoas muscle shadow is preserved, making psoas abscess unlikely and there is no evidence of a large soft tissue component. There is no evidence of fracture but a mild scoliosis is demonstrated at this level concave to the right.

The differential for these appearances in a young caucasian man includes:

- osteoid osteoma;
- osteoblastoma;
- healing fracture;
- sclerosing osteomyelitis (e.g. tuberculosis, syphilis);
- Brodie's abscess;
- osteoblastic metastasis;
- lymphoma;
- primary bone tumour (e.g. osteosarcoma).

Further radiological imaging is recommended and a choice needs to be made as to which modality will provide the best diagnostic yield with minimal inconvenience and radiation dose to this young patient. Considering the likely osseous location of the lesion, a computed tomography (CT) scan would have superior resolution compared to magnetic resonance imaging (MRI). Bone scintigraphy would also be beneficial but not as the first-line imaging modality following a plain film radiograph.

Figure 10.2 is a single axial slice of an unenhanced CT scan acquired at the level of the L4 vertebral body viewed with bone windows. Within the right pedicle there is a well-defined 17 mm lesion (arrow) that has a narrow zone of transition and is predominantly lytic in nature with some central calcification. There is diffuse sclerosis and expansion of the adjacent lamina and transverse process, with no evidence of periosteal reaction, spinal canal encroachment or pathological fracture. No soft tissue component is demonstrated. These features are in keeping with an osteoid osteoma, however considering its size (>15 mm) it is more appropriately described as an osteoblastoma.

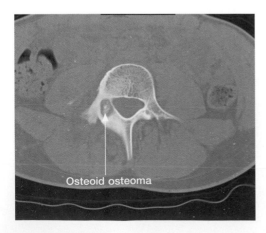

Osteoid osteoma

Figure 10.2 Unenhanced CT scan.

Osteoblastomas are rare benign tumours of the bone composed of multinucleated osteoclasts with irregular trabeculated bone and osteoid, surrounded by highly vascular fibrous connective tissue.[1] The commonest sites of involvement are around the knee joint in the long bones and within the posterior elements of the spine. They have unlimited potential for growth and carry a risk of malignant degeneration, therefore requiring definitive curative treatment at diagnosis.

The main treatment options include surgical removal, endovascular embolization, percutaneous CT-guided removal or percutaneous radiofrequency ablation. In this case, endovascular treatment was attempted (Figure 10.3).

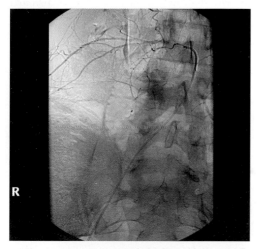

Figure 10.3 Angiographic image at embolization.

This angiographic image obtained at embolization (Figure 10.3) demonstrates a blush of contrast overlying the pedicle of the L4 vertebrae on selective cannulation of the right L4 lumbar artery. The arterial supply to this osteoblastoma was embolized with polyvinyl alcohol (PVA) and two microcoils. Follow-up 2 months later revealed an asymptomatic patient, and successful treatment was confirmed on CT with complete sclerosis at the site of the previous osteoblastoma (Figure 10.4).

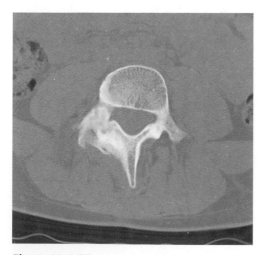

Figure 10.4 CT scan post embolization.

Reference

1. Dahnert, W. (2007) *Radiology Review Manual*, 6th edn. Philadelphia: Lippincott Williams and Wilkins.

History

You are asked to review a 67-year-old man in the chest clinic. He has been sent by his general practitioner (GP) who has been treating him for a cough. His symptoms started 3 weeks ago, at about the same time that the patient decided to stop smoking. The cough is chesty but non-productive, and is there constantly, but not worse, at night. He has no other new symptoms and is no more short of breath than usual, with an exercise tolerance of approximately 200 m. His appetite is unchanged and he has not lost weight. He does report occasional streaks of fresh red blood in the sputum on deep coughing.

The patient has a past medical history of excessive alcohol intake and chronic obstructive pulmonary disease (COPD). He had two previous admissions to hospital with decompensated liver disease, but has now abstained from alcohol for over a year. His last ultrasound scan confirms a degree of liver cirrhosis. He has smoked with a 60 pack-year history. He has never been admitted to intensive care with exacerbations of COPD, but has been treated for pneumonia in the past. He recently decided to stop smoking as his new girlfriend does not like to 'kiss an ashtray'.

Examination

As part of his management, the GP performed a chest radiograph (Figure 11.1) and then referred him to the chest clinic.

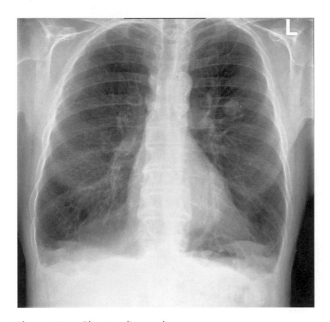

Figure 11.1 Chest radiograph.

Questions
- What does this chest radiograph demonstrate?
- What further radiological investigations are required?
- What is PET scanning?

This is a diagnostically adequate posterior–anterior (PA) chest radiograph of an adult male patient. There is a 2.3 cm rounded mass lesion within the left mid zone adjacent to the left hilum that appears to cavitate in its inferior aspect. No other pulmonary parenchymal nodularity is seen. There is blunting of the costophrenic angles bilaterally which may represent either small pleural effusions or be longstanding related to pleural thickening. There is a background of emphysematous change as evidenced by lung hyperinflation and flattening of the hemidiaphragms. Bilateral gynaecomastia is also noted. The rounded lesion may represent a malignancy in the form of a lung primary in view of the clinical history, however a focus of infection or metastasis cannot be excluded. Correlation with old films is advised.

The suspicious nature of this pulmonary mass lesion warrants a computed tomography (CT) scan, which ideally should be performed with intravenous contrast. Although the chest X-ray only demonstrates a solitary lesion, a CT scan of the chest and abdomen is recommended. This allows characterization of both the lungs and mediastinum, and also assesses the solid abdominal viscera (e.g. liver and adrenals), which are sites of common involvement in disseminated lung cancer. Extending the CT to involve the abdomen allows for accurate staging of primary lung cancer, and the patient can be referred to the lung multidisciplinary meeting (MDM) for further discussion.

The CT scan confirms a background of centrilobular emphysema and a left lower lobe pulmonary nodule measuring 2.6 × 1.6 cm (Figure 11.2). This tethers the oblique fissure and demonstrates an adjacent airspace opacification with cavitation. No disease was seen in the contralateral lung, mediastinum or below the diaphragm. Findings are compatible with a primary bronchial malignancy.

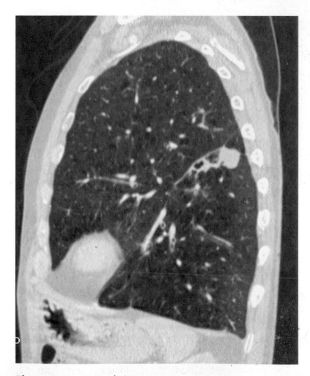

Figure 11.2 Sagittal CT scan.

The patient was then referred to the MDM. Time is an important factor to limit the spread of disease, and efficient transfer of patient care through the relevant specialities is of utmost importance to expedite definitive treatment.

A tissue diagnosis is important to obtain histological characterization of the lesion. Although cavitation and a history of smoking infers a likely squamous cell aetiology, histological confirmation is essential to tailor further chemotherapy or surgical treatment. The location of this lung primary would necessitate a CT-guided biopsy under the auspices of the interventional radiologists. A coaxial needle system is passed under CT guidance and local anaesthetic cover into the lesion, and a core biopsy sample taken (Figure 11.3). Patients should be consented for the risk of lung contusion and pneumothorax.

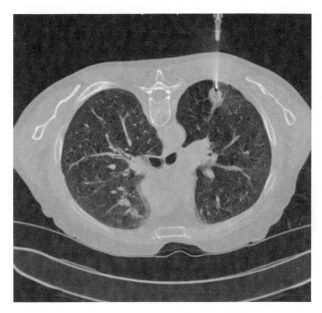

Figure 11.3 Biopsy under CT guidance.

A positron emission tomography (PET) scan is indicated in potentially operable tumours to assess nodal status and occult metastatic disease. This is required for complete disease staging and will dictate further treatment. If the PET scan confirms that this lesion is solitary and there is no evidence of nodal or metastatic spread, then the patient may be eligible for definitive surgery in the form of lobectomy if medically fit, although careful assessment will be needed in view of his significant COPD. Should the PET scan suggest inoperable or disseminated disease, then a chemotherapeutic treatment may be more appropriate.

A PET scan is a nuclear medicine scan, usually performed in combination with a CT scan. PET uses a radioactive isotope with a short half-life (e.g. fluorine-18 (F^{18})), which is biochemically incorporated into the functionally active glucose molecule fluorodeoxyglucose (FDG). It is used extensively in oncology imaging because the FDG–F^{18} is concentrated in metabolically active tissues, radiolabelling those tissues with high amounts of glucose uptake. Although there is physiological uptake in organs such as the brain, heart and liver, primary cancers and their metastases can also be detected by the PET scanner, as the F^{18} undergoes positron emission decay. The images obtained are fused with unenhanced, attenuation corrected CT images taken concurrently for anatomical correlation.

Although not its primary function, CT can also allow further detection and assessment of both related and unrelated pathology. As well as primary staging, PET scanning can be used to assess response to treatment. Despite being an effective tool, its major limitations are related to cost (both of the scanner and in generating the isotope) and lesion size: small metastases (<1 cm) may not accumulate detectable levels of FDG-F^{18}.

 KEY POINTS

- A patient with a chest radiograph suspicious for lung cancer should be referred for a chest CT scan to characterize the lesion further.
- Lung biopsy can be performed under CT guidance for histological characterization.
- A PET scan is often used to assess suitability when planning the treatment for a patient with lung cancer.

CASE 12: A SCHOOLMASTER WITH PROGRESSIVE BREATHLESSNESS

History

A 64-year-old man is referred to the respiratory outpatient clinic for assessment. He gives a history of a shortness of breath which has been insidious in onset over the last 4 years. Over the last year, this has been associated with a dry cough which he cannot seem to clear despite several courses of antibiotics. He feels fatigued and had found it more difficult to complete a round of golf, which he used to do twice a week. His weight has remained steady and he denies orthopnoea. There is no relevant past medical history. He is a non-smoker and admits to social drinking only. He takes 75 mg aspirin daily on advice of his general practitioner (GP) but is not on any other regular medication. Occupationally, he is nearing retirement as a school headmaster and denies any history of occupational dust exposure. He lives at home with his wife and keeps no pets.

Examination

On examination, he is well perfused and not cyanosed, but has evidence of nail clubbing bilaterally. Lung expansion is reduced and auscultation demonstrates fine inspiratory crackles, more marked at the bases.

Prearranged lung function studies demonstrate a restrictive lung defect and a chest radiograph was taken for assessment (Figure 12.1).

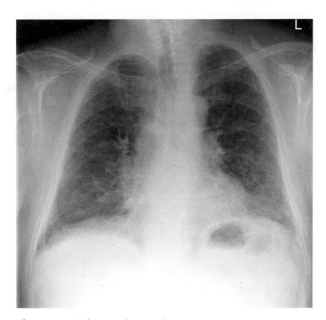

Figure 12.1 Chest radiograph.

Questions

- How would you describe the chest radiograph appearances?
- What would be the differential for these appearances?
- How is the idiopathic cause of this condition subclassified?

ANSWER 12

This is a posterior–anterior (PA) chest radiograph of an adult male patient. There is good alignment, inspiration and penetration. The heart and hila are of normal size with an ill-defined 'shaggy' heart boarder. The lungs demonstrate volume loss, most marked at the bases with depression of the horizontal fissure on the right. There is reticular shadowing to the lung parenchyma in a subpleural distribution with relative sparing of the apices. There is no evidence of calcified lymph nodes or air–fluid levels within the oesophagus. Correlation with old radiographs is recommended, but the appearances are suggestive of pulmonary fibrosis.

Many people have difficulty with the descriptive terms of 'reticular' and 'nodular' shadowing. They are commonly used in chest radiograph reporting, implying clear differentials and distinction between infective and interstitial causes of lung disease. Reticulation describes lines that branch and interlace as a result of thickened interstitial septa between secondary pulmonary lobules. Nodularity, however, describes well-defined 'dots', which can vary in size and are predominantly caused by airspace opacification and imply an infective focus. Just to confuse matters, some conditions (e.g. sarcoidosis) can be both reticular and nodular in appearance.

In this scenario, the reticular pattern implies an underlying diagnosis of interstitial lung disease, with volume loss suggesting a fibrotic component. The causes of these appearances are numerous, and it is important to scrutinize the distribution of disease to help narrow the differential. The causes of lung fibrosis, divided between an apical and basal distribution, are listed in Table 12.1.

Table 12.1 Causes of lung fibrosis

Upper zone fibrosis	Lower zone fibrosis
Allergic bronchopulmonary aspergillosis	Idiopathic pulmonary fibrosis
Radiation	Drugs (e.g. amiodarone)
Extrinsic allergic alveolitis	Rheumatoid disease
Ankylosing spondylitis	Scleroderma
Sarcoidosis	Asbestosis
Silicosis	Dermatomyosytis
Tuberculosis	
Histocytosis X	

By history alone and in the absence of ancillary features associated with connective tissue disease, a diagnosis of idiopathic pulmonary fibrosis is made in this patient. To confirm and subclassify the diagnosis, the patient should be referred for a high-resolution computed tomography (HRCT) chest scan. This is different from a normal 'volume' computed tomography (CT) scan of the chest and is an unenhanced study, providing high-resolution thin (1 mm) cuts of the lung parenchyma at 1 cm intervals (Figure 12.2).

This single image of the patient's HRCT obtained within the lower zones of the chest demonstrates areas of disruption to the normal lung parenchyma with thickening of the interlobular septa causing a 'honeycomb' like appearance. These changes are predominantly confined to a subpleural distribution with preservation of the normal lung parenchyma centrally. This is characteristic of usual interstitial pneumonitis (UIP), a subtype of idiopathic pulmonary fibrosis. There is clinical importance in determining the likely subtype, as UIP is relatively insensitive to steroid therapy with a 45 per cent 5-year mortality.[1] The other broad subtypes are:

- **Non-specific interstitial pneumonitis (NSIP):** Despite an often normal chest radiograph, appearances on HRCT are of patchy ground glass opacification with no clear zonal distribution. There is no evidence of honeycomb fibrosis and this subtype is more likely to respond to steroid therapy with an overall 5-year mortality of 11 per cent.[1]
- **Desquamative interstitial pneumonitis (DIP):** Seen predominantly in patients who smoke, appearances on chest radiograph and HRCT are of both subpleural ground glass opacification and honeycomb fibrosis. This is confined to the lower zones but is not associated with significant volume loss. DIP has a variable steroid response with a 50 per cent 5-year survival.[1]

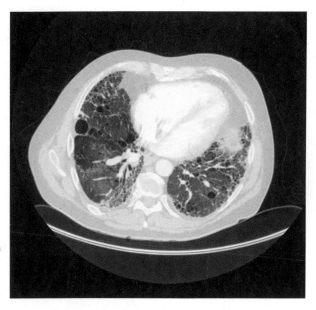

Figure 12.2 High resolution chest CT scan.

KEY POINTS

- Reticular shadowing with parenchymal volume loss is the characteristic feature of pulmonary fibrosis on chest radiograph.
- It is important to scrutinise the distribution of disease within the lungs to help make the causative diagnosis.
- HRCT is integral in characterizing the type and extent of pulmonary fibrosis.

Reference

1. Dahnert, W. (2007) *Radiology Review Manual*, 6th edn. Philadelphia: Lippincott Williams and Wilkins.

History

A 50-year-old man presents with a history of an intermittently numb right arm that has become more of a problem recently after some heavy lifting. There is no history of trauma or surgery and there is no clear history of onset although the problem has been present for some months. He notices it most after sleeping, with forearm and hand numbness that wears off with movement. He also has an intermittent dull ache and impression of reduced strength, for example when trying to open jars. There is no history of Raynaud's phenomenon, swelling or cold hand. There is no other significant medical history.

Examination

The arms are symmetrical. There are normal peripheral pulses. There is a subjective mild weakness on the right to flexion at the elbow with a slightly reduced biceps reflex. Reflexes and sensation are otherwise normal. No pulse changes are noted in hyperabduction or on deep inspiration with the head turned to the right side (Adson's manoeuvre). In the right supraclavicular fossa a small hard lesion is palpable. The chest and abdomen are normal.

You arrange a chest radiograph (Figure 13.1a,b).

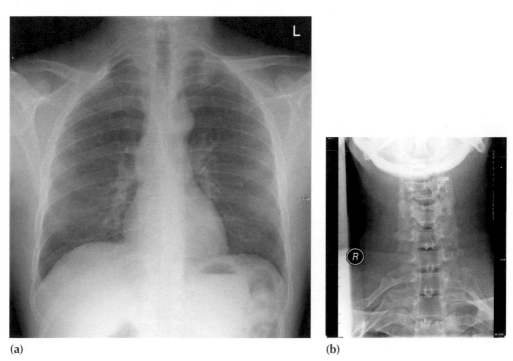

(a)   (b)

Figure 13.1 (a) Chest and (b) anterior–posterior (AP) cervical spine radiographs.

Questions

• What differential diagnoses are you considering?
• What does the radiograph show?
• What imaging or investigation would you do next?

The differential diagnosis for this presentation is quite broad and can be narrowed down in broad classes. The symptoms are predominantly neurological and primary neurological causes such as spinal stenosis, tumour, cerebral infarct or multiple sclerosis or secondary causes including thoracic outlet syndrome affecting the brachial plexus, ulnar nerve compression and carpal tunnel syndrome should be considered. The possible weakness of elbow flexion and biceps reflex suggests a C5/C6 level lesion. There is less evidence for a vascular cause such as Raynaud's disease, vasculitis or vascular compression. Other causes include trauma and soft tissue lesions such as a Pancoast tumour.

The radiograph shows bilateral cervical ribs. The mediastinum and lungs appear normal. The right cervical rib has a pseudoarthrosis (false joint) in the mid portion that corresponds with the hard palpable lesion in the supraclavicular fossa.

Although a vascular cause seems unlikely, an angiogram – selective imaging of vessels – may be helpful to check for compression of the subclavian vessels. Arteries or veins can be selectively studied by injection of contrast either by direct catheterization in combination with fluoroscopy, or intravenous injection and selective timing of the computed tomography (CT) scan. A catheter angiogram rather than a CT angiogram allows the patient to be put in different positions to try to induce the intermittent symptoms. The angiogram in Figure 13.2a proved to be normal. Given the predominantly neurological symptoms, further imaging should concentrate on identifying the position of the underlying lesion best done with magnetic resonance (MR) to examine soft tissue and nerve roots at the cervical spine and brachial plexus (Figure 13.2b). MR is less sensitive for cortical bone and a cervical spine radiograph for comparison is also helpful.

The patient's symptoms are caused by the disc prolapse (demonstrated on MR) rather than thoracic outlet syndrome due to the cervical ribs.

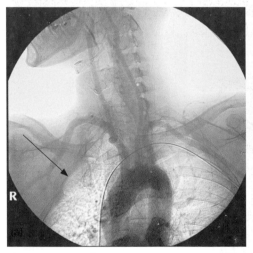 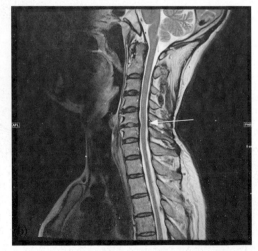

Figure 13.2 (a) Fluoroscopic arteriogram. The arrow shows displacement but no compression of the right subclavian artery. (b) T2-weighted sagittal MR image showing degenerative changes at C5/6 with disc protrusion into the canal (arrow) also resulting in nerve root compression.

🔑 KEY POINTS

- Thoracic outlet syndrome can be subdivided into neurological, arterial and venous causes. The symptoms may help decide the most likely cause.
- Cervical ribs are a fairly common finding and often asymptomatic.

History

A 41-year-old woman attended hospital for an ultrasound appointment requested by her general practitioner (GP). She had undergone a laparoscopic cholecystectomy 4 months previously and had recovered well, but over the last 3 weeks she had been complaining of increasing pain in the right upper quadrant and occasional itching. She denied any weight loss or jaundice, and reported normal appearances to her stool and urine. She is a non-drinker with no other notable medical history.

Examination

On examination she had slightly icteric sclera. She was comfortable at rest but had scratch marks on her upper arms from recent itching. The cardiovascular and respiratory examinations were normal, and her abdomen was soft with slight tenderness of the right upper quadrant on deep palpation. There was no organomegaly.

Investigations showed a normal full blood count and renal function, but liver function showed an elevated bilirubin and alkaline phosphatase with normal transaminases and albumin levels. Her amylase was normal.

She was referred for an abdominal ultrasound to assess her liver parenchyma (Figures 14.1 and 14.2).

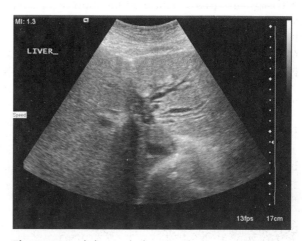

Figure 14.1 Abdominal ultrasound.

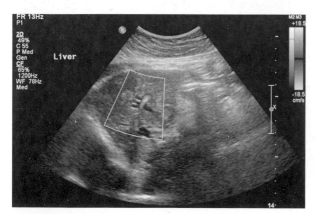

Figure 14.2

Questions

- What does the ultrasound demonstrate?
- What procedure is performed in Figure 14.2?
- What is interventional radiology?

Figure 14.1 is a single ultrasound image of the left lobe of the liver obtained with a curvilinear transducer (C5–2) in a longitudinal orientation. The liver appears of normal echogenicity and echo texture with a smooth capsular contour. No focal lesion is seen on this image. There are anechoic linear structures seen which extend to the periphery with a maximal diameter of 4 mm, and colour Doppler assessment in Figure 14.2 demonstrates no flow within them. This is in keeping with intrahepatic biliary duct dilatation, and the remainder of the study did not demonstrate an obstructing lesion although the common bile duct (CBD) was 7 mm in diameter, which is within normal limits for a patient post cholecystectomy. The patient was referred for a liver magnetic resonance imaging (MRI) scan for further characterization. The liver function tests of raised bilirubin and alkaline phosphatase with normal transaminases and albumin suggest obstruction with normal cellular and synthetic function.

Figure 14.3 is a coronal maximal intensity projection (MIP) image of the same patient acquired from heavily T2-weighted sequences. It confirms moderate intrahepatic biliary duct dilatation and also demonstrates a focal tapered stenosis at the level of the common hepatic duct. There is no intraductal filling defect or stenosing soft tissue mass lesion, and the CBD and pancreatic duct are of normal calibre. The appearances suggest a stricture of the common hepatic duct which may be ischaemic, post inflammatory or neoplastic in nature. Endoscopic retrograde cholangiopancreatography (ERCP) was advised to obtain cytology brushings, attempt to correct the obstruction and decompress the intrahepatic ducts, but a stent could not be inserted. The patient was therefore referred to the interventional radiology department for a percutaneous transhepatic cholangiogram (PTC).

The single image of the PTC (Figure 14.4) was acquired by opacifying the intrahepatic ducts with radiographic contrast during a fluoroscopy procedure. The dilated ducts of the left system were punctured under ultrasound guidance, and a guidewire was then manipulated across the hilar stricture and down into the duodenum. A sheath (8F) was inserted to stabilize the position, and contrast was injected through this to perform the cholangiogram. A stent can be passed over the wire and placed across the stenosis to relieve the obstruction and improve patient symptoms. This procedure is performed by the interventional radiology department.

Interventional radiology (IR) is an expanding subspeciality of radiology that uses imaging guidance and minimally invasive techniques to diagnose and treat a patient. A trained radiologist uses their experience in ultrasound, computed tomography (CT) and fluoroscopy to guide the passage of a needle or catheter to a site of interest and perform a task that would otherwise be surgically difficult and involve significant morbidity in the form of an open operation. Interventional radiology consultants can use the veins, arteries and biliary ducts to access deep or distal lesions, vessels or organs, often leaving only a pinhole size scar at the site of puncture (often the groin) as a sign of recent treatment. This allows tissue conservation, reduced morbidity and faster recovery for patients. The scope of the speciality is too broad to be effectively covered in this answer, but the procedures used include the following:

- Angiography: A vein or artery can be punctured with ultrasound guidance, and contrast is injected mapping the vessel anatomy under fluoroscopy. Stenoses and occlusions can be characterized and an expandable balloon is used to improve blood flow. This is termed 'angioplasty'.

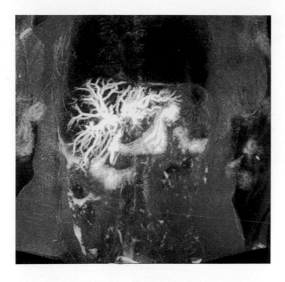

Figure 14.3 Coronal maximal intensity projection image.

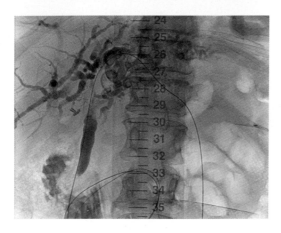

Figure 14.4 Percutaneous transhepatic cholangiogram.

- **Biopsy:** Ultrasound (superficial lesions) and CT (complicated or deep lesions) can help to guide a needle accurately to a lesion of interest for core biopsy and histological characterization.
- **Drainage:** Inserting a drain can offer a conduit for decompression of infected collections or uncomfortable ascites. Optimal and accurate placement is obtained by imaging guidance.
- **Stenting:** Expandable stents can be inserted into a vessel or duct to act as 'scaffolding' and can exert radial force to maintain patency in atherosclerosis or tumour stenosis.
- **Line insertion:** Patients on long-term therapy (e.g. dialysis, antibiotics, chemotherapy) require definitive vascular access (e.g. Hickman line, portacath) to avoid the discomfort of recurrent peripheral cannulation and thrombophlebitis.
- **Embolization:** Instilling an embolic agent (coils, particles or glue) into a selectively cannulated vessel can control active haemorrhage, prevent aneurismal rupture or infarct a tumour (e.g. uterine fibroid). An adjunct to this is chemoembolization, where a chemotherapy agent is instilled directly to a tumour and then the blood vessel is embolized to cause tumour infarction.

- **Radiofrequency ablation:** Small malignant lesions can be cauterized via a specialized electrical probe that is inserted under image guidance for accurate placement.
- **Vertebroplasty:** Guiding the infusion of inert cement into a collapsed spinal vertebra can provide stability in cases of osteoporotic or metastatic collapse.

 KEY POINTS

- Ultrasound is excellent for the assessment of the liver and has a high sensitivity for detecting intrahepatic biliary duct dilatation.
- Biliary obstruction can be circumvented by stent insertion either via ERCP or PTC.
- Interventional radiology is a subspeciality of radiology that uses image guidance to perform minimally invasive techniques.

CASE 15: INFANT WITH CLICKING HIPS

History

A 6-week-old female infant is brought by her mother as part of the 6-week check in general practice. The baby was delivered at term by caesarian section due to a breech presentation. Her maternal grandmother and aunt are known to have chronic hip problems.

Examination

On examination she moves both lower limbs normally. The hip creases appear a little asymmetric. On Barlow's manoeuvre (adduction of the hip with light pressure on the knee) the right hip appears to pop posteriorly and then anteriorly on Ortolani's manoeuvre (the hips and knees are flexed to 90 degrees and anterior pressure is applied to the greater trochanters while using the thumbs to abduct the legs).

You expedite the hip ultrasound that has already been arranged due to the risk factors (Figure 15.1).

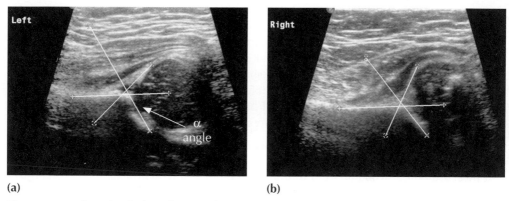

(a)   (b)

Figure 15.1 Left and right hip ultrasound images (coronal flexion view).

Questions

- Who gets hip ultrasound?
- What do the images in Figure 15.1 show?
- Is a radiograph helpful?
- What happens next?

Hip ultrasound is done on neonates and young infants (<6 months) to screen or check for developmental dysplasia of the hip. Screening is done on infants with risk factors that include family history, breech presentation, foot deformities or neuromuscular disorders. Examination features that raise suspicion for hip abnormality include asymmetric groin creases, a click on movement and a click or subluxation on provocation tests.

As with all ultrasound, gel is used to couple the ultrasound beam into the soft tissue and allow movement of the probe without loss of image. The baby is placed in the lateral position with the hip flexed and the probe is placed parallel to the ilium (bright line on the left of the image) and the orientation optimized to produce a horizontal image like a golf ball (stippled cartilage of the femoral head) on a tee (cup is the acetebulum, stalk is the ilium). If the golf ball appears to be falling off the tee (upwards on the image), then the femoral head is subluxed and the acetabular cup is shallow. This is all formalized by measuring angles (indicated on the image). The alpha angle measures the acetabular roof angle with the ilium and normally measures over 60 degrees. The beta angle assesses the prominence of the labrum (cartilaginous flange around the acetabulum).

Figure 15.1 shows a normal left hip but a low alpha angle (53.5 degrees) on the right, corresponding with a shallow acetabulum and hip instability. The ultrasound shows a lot of soft tissue detail, including the unossified cartilage as well as the bone, although the anterior bone edge blocks the beam and no deeper structure is seen. Plain radiographs complement this view by demonstrating the bone structure but with very poor soft tissue detail. Ultrasound is the investigation of choice in infants with unossified femoral heads but as the ossification centre develops and blocks the ultrasound from about 6 months onwards, radiographs are more useful. Figure 15.2 shows the hip radiograph at 4 months.

The aim is to diagnose a hip abnormality as soon as possible to minimize the degree of intervention required to fix the problem. Treatment ranges from observing (if very mild and picked up on a neonatal scan) to braces or surgical intervention.

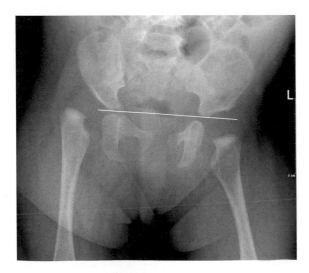

Figure 15.2 Radiograph at 4 months with right hip subluxation and a shallow right acetabulum (relative to Hilgenreiner's line drawn on the radiograph).

	KEY POINTS

- Ultrasound is the method of choice for examining infant hips.
- Hip screening in infants with family history or breech presentation occurs at 4–6 weeks.

History

A 13-year-old girl presents to the accident and emergency department with a painful right wrist after falling while roller skating. She fell backwards with her arm outstretched. Her wrist appears deformed, but she tells you that although it hurts, the wrist has had that appearance for a long time and that it was investigated at another hospital many years ago. She gives a family history of bone problems but is otherwise well with no medical problems.

Examination

On the volar aspect of the right forearm just proximal to the wrist there is a firm swelling that extends laterally. There is some associated tenderness but no malalignment of the wrist or hand. There is normal movement, pulses and sensation. The chest and abdomen are normal. Given the history you also briefly examine the arms and spine that appear normal and the legs. The bone around the knees is prominent, with an asymptomatic bony nodule over the lateral aspect of the proximal right tibia.

You arrange radiographs of the arm (Figure 16.1a,b).

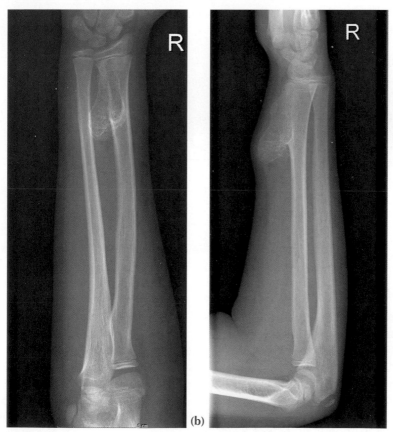

(a) (b)

Figure 16.1 Anterior–posterior (AP) and lateral radiographs.

Questions

- What do the radiographs show?
- Can you name some differential diagnoses?
- What other imaging should be obtained?

ANSWER 16

The radiographs show a lobulated expansile lesion arising from the cortical bone of the radial metaphysis and extending proximally. The bone is well delineated with a narrow zone of transition, an appearance suggesting the lesion is benign. No fracture is seen.

The appearance is in keeping with an exostosis, also known as an osteochondroma, that results from dysplasia of the growth plate. This may be solitary or multiple in a condition known as multiple hereditary exostosis (or diaphyseal aclasis), or rarely as part of various syndromes such as Turner's syndrome or tuberous sclerosis.

Rather than take more images of the arm, the best course of action would be to obtain previous images. Picture archiving and communication system (PACS) is the digital system developed to manage the images primarily produced in hospital radiology departments. In the last decade it has almost entirely replaced film-based archives with the advantages of rapid search and comparison, remote and web-based access and integration into other hospital information systems. In this patient, a previous skeletal image on PACS (Figure 16.2) suggests the diagnosis of multiple hereditary exostosis.

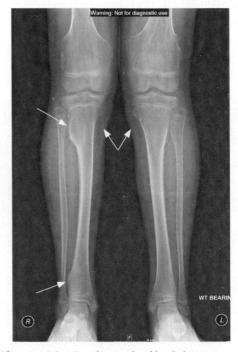

Figure 16.2 AP radiograph of both legs showing large right proximal and distal lateral tibial exostoses and bilateral proximal medial tibial exostoses (see arrows).

Multiple hereditary exostosis is inherited as an autosomal dominant trait, with an incidence of about 1 in 50000. Children are diagnosed on average around 3 years old. As seen in this case, bony growths (exostoses) arise from the metaphyses, point away from epiphysis, and extend down the diaphysis during growth. They increase in size and number with age, arising in several characteristic sites. Over 90 per cent of cases are at the distal and proximal tibia, proximal femur and proximal humerus. Ribs, scapula, radius, ulna, ilium and phalanges are also common sites.

Clinical complications include trauma and fractures, particularly at exposed positions at the wrist and knees. The exostosis may exert pressure on surrounding soft tissue and cause neurovascular compromise. There can be inequality in limb length or short stature. In a small proportion of patients (1–2 per cent) at a later age (>21) an exostosis undergoes sarcomatous transformation into a chondrosarcoma. This is more likely in exostoses of the pelvis, scapula, proximal humerus, proximal femur and spine, and may be associated with a change in size or onset of pain.

🔑 **KEY POINTS**

- Exostoses can be solitary or multiple and develop from the metaphysis while the growth plate is open.
- Exostoses can cause symptoms. In older symptomatic patients, malignant transformation should be considered although it is uncommon.

History

A 78-year-old woman presents to the oncology clinic with a 1 week history of right upper quadrant and epigastric tenderness and constipation for 3 days. She has a history of metastatic ovarian cancer treated with abdominal hysterectomy, oophorectomy and omentectomy for peritoneal disease 15 months ago. She has also had chemotherapy. On her last scan she was noted to have lung nodules, mediastinal and mesenteric lymph node enlargement that appeared stable and a new caecal metastatic deposit.

Examination

On examination, she is not acutely unwell. Her observations are normal. The chest and heart sound normal. The upper abdomen is tender and there is a palpable fullness or mass below the right costophrenic margin.

You assess an abdominal radiograph (Figure 17.1) during clinic and decide to admit the patient for assessment and a computed tomography (CT) scan.

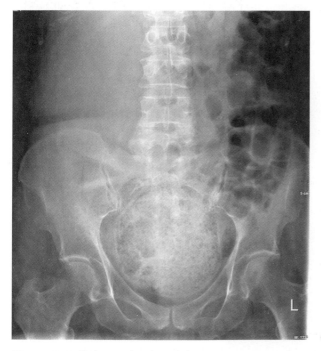

Figure 17.1 Abdominal radiograph.

Questions
- What is the likely cause of her pain?
- What does the radiograph show?
- What appearance do bowel contents have?

Based on the history of cancer and surgery, the patient is at risk of bowel obstruction secondary to adhesions associated with surgery or tumour infiltration. Metastatic ovarian carcinoma frequently metastasizes through the peritoneal space, seeding deposits onto the omentum (removed in this patient's case) and mesentery. Liver metastases are also possible, causing pain from stretching the liver capsule, biliary obstruction or ascites. Other common causes that are less likely in this case are cholecystitis and appendicitis.

The radiograph shows a large volume of faeces in the pelvis within large bowel or rectum and gas-filled empty bowel loops on the left side of the abdomen. There is a paucity of bowel gas on the right together with impression of a large soft tissue region extending throughout the right side of the abdomen. Small bowel can be distinguished from large by its central position and a fold pattern likened to a coiled spring (valvulae conniventes) less than 3 cm in normal diameter. Large bowel tends to frame the abdomen with haustral folds that are widely spaced and not circumferential (i.e. they do not cross the whole diameter of the visible bowel).

The patient's CT (Figure 17.2) shows a large right upper quadrant mass, probably a metastatic deposit, displacing empty transverse colon to the left and partially obstructing the caecum that is distended by faeces. Gallstones are also seen; these are not apparent on the plain radiograph.

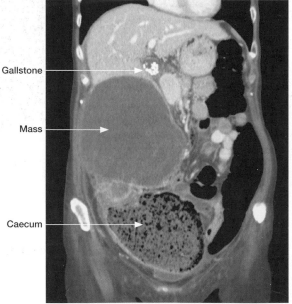

Gallstone

Mass

Caecum

Figure 17.2 Reconstructed coronal CT slice of the abdomen and pelvis.

The colon receives the sterile dilute product of digestion and then proceeds to remove a large proportion of the fluid content as well as employing microbial digestion (fermentation) to extract various products not produced in small bowel digestion, such as vitamin K. As a result, faeces take on a more solid appearance as they move round the colon. In addition, the microbial activity produces gas and the stool has a characteristic foamy appearance. Stomach contents also have a similar appearance with food mixed with fluid and air. Small bowel tends to be predominantly homogeneously fluid filled in appearance although with a small amount of gas that increases if there is obstruction.

KEY POINTS

- The distribution of stool tends to be of more significance than its appearance.
- Constipation may be indicated by a large volume of stool throughout the bowel, a rather solid appearance to the stool in the rectum or impacted faeces above an obstruction.
- Radiographs are rarely indicated for constipation unless obstruction is suspected.

History

A 30-year-old man presents to you with a chronic history of headache that has worsened significantly in the last week. Investigations for the same problem 9 months ago ruled out sinus disease. He is concerned that this may be due to a brain tumour. Several relatives have died of various types of cancer. There is no history of definite head trauma, although he has had various sporting injuries. There is no other history of significant illness. On careful questioning the headache is reported to be present on waking and worsens on coughing.

Examination

On examination he is well. His observations are normal. There is papilloedema on examination of the eyes but no focal neurology is demonstrated. Examination is otherwise normal.

You arrange a computed tomography (CT) scan of the head.

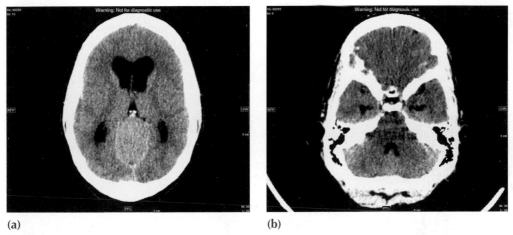

(a) (b)

Figure 18.1 Axial CT image of the brain at the level of (a) the third ventricle and (b) the fourth ventricle.

Questions

- Headache is a common problem. What red flag symptoms help to decide on investigations?
- What does the CT show?
- What would you do next?

Headache is a common problem, often assessed in general practice and often associated with tumours by patients. The annual incidence of brain tumours is about 10 per 100 000 per year whereas up to 4000 per 100 000 GP consultations are for headache, so some discrimination has to be used to avoid imaging every patient.

If you see papilloedema then red flags are not required, urgent investigation is mandatory, after checking your records for previous investigation – very occasionally it is idiopathic and chronic. More commonly, fundoscopy is not performed well enough to see changes. Other red flags include:

- systemic symptoms (e.g. neck stiffness) or secondary risk factors (e.g. cancer, HIV, thrombosis);
- neurological symptoms or signs;
- onset (e.g. thunderclap headache);
- new progressive or unilateral headache in older patients (consider temporal arteritis);
- previous headache history changing pattern;
- triggered headache (e.g. cough, sneeze, straining).

The CT shows a large midline mass in the region of the pineal gland extending into the subtentorial region, displacing the cerebellar vermis and hemispheres inferiorly and compressing the aqueduct and fourth ventricle. There is dilatation of the lateral and third ventricles but undilated fourth ventricle and basal cisterns in keeping with obstructive hydrocephalus.

The next step is to characterize the midline lesion using magnetic resonance (MR) (Figure 18.2). This confirms hydrocephalus caused by a pineal fossa or tectal plate mass with evidence of cerebrospinal fluid (CSF) in the periventricular tissue, suggesting the obstruction is acute. The lesion may be a pineoblastoma.

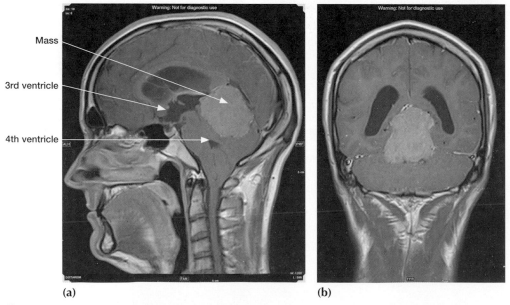

(a)   **(b)**

Figure 18.2 (a) Coronal and (b) midline sagittal T1 MR sequence images after gadolinium contrast.

Hydrocephalus appears on scans as dilated CSF spaces and can be caused by obstruction, as in this case. Communicating hydrocephalus occurs in the absence of obstruction due to overproduction of CSF (e.g. tumour), defective absorption of CSF (most common, e.g. after haemorrhage) or venous drainage insufficiency. Normal pressure hydrocephalus occurs in older patients characterized by dilatation but no elevation of CSF pressure at lumbar puncture and may be caused by intermittent intracranial hypertension.

This patient requires referral to a neurosurgical centre as the hydrocephalus requires acute treatment with a shunt, as well as treatment planning for the underlying tumour.

 KEY POINTS

- Headache is a common symptom and is only rarely caused by a brain tumour.
- Hydrocephalus can be acute or chronic, communicating or obstructive.
- CT is the initial investigation for acute neurological problems to check for haemorrhage, hydrocephalus and presence of mass lesions.

CASE 19: PERSISTENT COUGH

History

A 65-year-old woman with a persistent cough comes to see you in general practice. She says that the cough has been present for months but that it has got worse in the last week with associated coryzal symptoms. There is no history of haemoptysis, chest pain or weight loss. She does not have asthma and is on medication for high blood pressure and high cholesterol. She has a 30 pack-year smoking history, although she gave up 2 years ago.

Examination

There is no abnormality on examination of the respiratory system. Temperature and pulse are normal; her blood pressure is 136/82. There is no significant neck lymphadenopathy or tonsillar enlargement.

You consider the diagnosis of an acute upper respiratory tract infection with a background persistent cough. The cough has not been investigated before and you explain to the patient that you will arrange a chest X-ray (Figure 19.1) but that antibiotics do not seem appropriate currently.

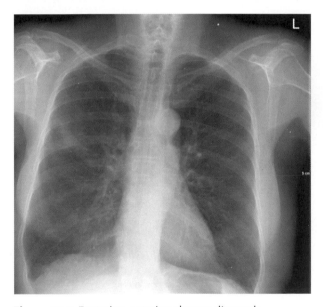

Figure 19.1 Posterior–anterior chest radiograph.

Questions
- What does the radiograph show?
- What are the most likely diagnoses?
- What is the next step?

ANSWER 19

The radiograph shows a single spiculated mass in the right mid zone. No significant hilar or mediastinal widening is seen.

The differential diagnosis for a single pulmonary mass includes primary or secondary carcinoma, hamartoma (especially if fat and calcification can be identified), pneumonia or arteriovenous malformation. The patient's age, smoking history and chronic cough are red flags for considering carcinoma.

The next step is rapid referral of the patient to chest clinic with a preceding staging computed tomography (CT) scan. Most hospitals have a streamlined process for the radiology department to flag up the patient to the relevant specialist clinic if cancer is suspected, in anticipation of an urgent general practitioner (GP) referral.

The diagnosis of non-small cell lung carcinoma and stage of disease was confirmed by biopsy and positron emission tomography (PET) scan that confirmed T2a (<5 cm) N0 M0 (no affected lymph nodes or metastases) staging. The tumour was removed with the right upper lobe (lobectomy).

The post-lobectomy radiograph (Figure 19.2a) shows signs of loss of right lung volume with elevation of the right hemidiaphragm and hilum but no significant right rib space narrowing.

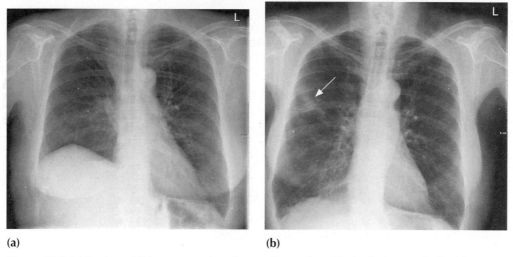

(a)   (b)

Figure 19.2 (a) Post- and (b) pre-operative chest radiographs with the lesion marked with an arrow.

GPs have access to many imaging modalities at their local hospital, although plain radiographs and ultrasound are the most used. They receive copies of the image reports, typically within a week, but are not able to view the images. The Royal College of Radiologists has produced referral guidelines.[1]

Chronic cough is a common GP presentation. The British Thoracic Society has produced guidelines on how to manage chronic cough,[2] a chest radiograph being one of the first steps. Subsequent imaging depends on the diagnosis and whether imaging is likely to be helpful in management.

KEY POINTS

- Pulmonary lobectomy results in loss of volume with possible elevation of the hemidiaphragm and hilum, rib crowding or little or no volume change with hyperexpansion of the residual lobes with associated increased translucency.
- GPs have access to imaging modalities but typically do not have access to the images and therefore it is important that the request states the clinical context and question and the report provides an answer.

Reference

1. Royal College of Radiologists (2007) *Making the Best Use of Clinical Radiology Services*, 6th edn. London: Royal College of Radiologists.
2. British Thoracic Society (2006) Recommendations for the Management of Cough in Adults. Produced by British Thoracic Society Cough Guideline Group; a sub-committee of the Standards of Care Committee of the British Thoracic Society. *Thorax* 61(suppl 1): i1–i24.

CASE 20: CHEST PAIN AND DYSPNOEA

History

This 66-year-old woman was referred to the accident and emergency department by her general practitioner (GP) with a 2 week history of dyspnoea, cough and fever that has been worsening and an unclear history of new onset pleuritic chest pain. There is also a history of a chronic pressure sore, type 2 diabetes and high blood pressure treated with appropriate medication. The GP had treated her for a few days with antibiotics initially with little effect.

Examination

Her temperature is 39.3°C, pulse 104/minute, oxygen saturation 89 per cent breathing air and there appears to be a right ventricular heave. There are coarse lung sounds in the right upper zone posteriorly. The abdomen is soft and non-tender. The left hip is painful but demonstrates normal range of movement and weight bearing. There is a mild degree of peripheral sensory neuropathy but the legs are otherwise normal.

You arrange tests including a chest radiograph (Figure 20.1).

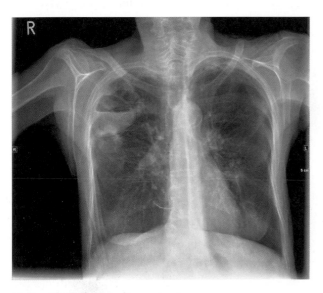

Figure 20.1 Chest radiograph.

Questions

- What does the chest radiograph show?
- What are possible causes of the abnormality?

There is one and possibly a second circular cavitating lesion in the right upper zone that contains an air–fluid level and has a thin wall superiorly. There is bilateral apical thickening. The hila appear normal and the heart is not enlarged. A displaced old fracture of the left clavicle is noted.

There are multiple causes of cavities in the lung and features that help decide on likely differential diagnoses include the clinical context, number of lesions, wall thickness, appearance of contents (if any), position and presence of enlarged lymph nodes.

In terms of categories, cavities may form due to:

- infection, such as *Staphylococcus* (frequently multiple), *Klebsiella*, tuberculosis (frequently associated with fibrosis) and aspiration (these cavities are usually thick walled and may contain fluid levels);
- neoplasm, such as bronchogenic carcinoma (particularly squamous cell carcinoma, SCC), metastases such as SCC, colon and sarcoma, Hodgkin's disease (with lymphadenopathy), often with thick walls;
- vascular infarction that may cavitate or become infected and cavitate;
- trauma, either the result of a haematoma or formation of a traumatic lung cyst;
- abnormal lung – infected emphysematous bulla;
- cavitating nodular vasculitic disease such as Wegener's granulomatosis, rheumatoid arthritis and occasionally granulomatous disease such as sarcoidosis, which all frequently have multiple cavities.

Given the patient's tachycardia, ventricular heave and hypoxia it is also important to consider cardiac causes and possible pulmonary embolism. A computed tomography (CT) pulmonary angiogram was arranged (Figure 20.2a,b).

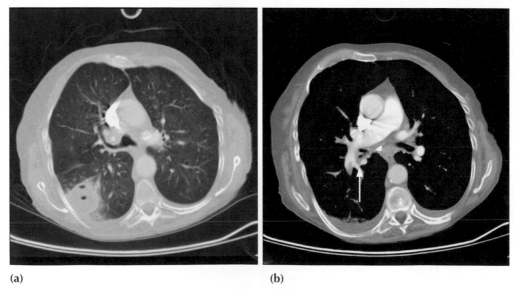

(a) (b)

Figure 20.2 CT pulmonary angiogram showing a right lower lobe fluid-filled cavity (a) and, on the slice just inferior (b), a pulmonary embolus in the right lower lobe pulmonary artery (white arrow).

The most likely differential diagnoses are cavitation and infection secondary to an embolus or a cavitating lung malignancy with secondary pulmonary embolus. The short history and fever suggest infection and the subsequent course showed that the former diagnosis was correct.

 KEY POINTS

- Position, number of lesions, wall thickness and contents may be helpful in determining the cause of lung cavities.
- Cavities are potential sites for secondary infection.

History

This 17-year-old man presents to his GP with a swelling at the base of his neck that he noticed recently after swimming. He also complains of tiredness, some loss of appetite and night sweats developing over the last 4–6 weeks. There is no other medical history. He has not travelled outside Europe and is not aware of recent exposure to any infectious disease.

Examination

On examination he has normal weight and does not appear unwell. He has normal observations. There is a palpable mass in the left supraclavicular fossa and prominent nodes in the neck and axillae. The chest is clear. The abdomen is soft and not tender. You take blood tests and arrange for a chest radiograph (Figure 21.1).

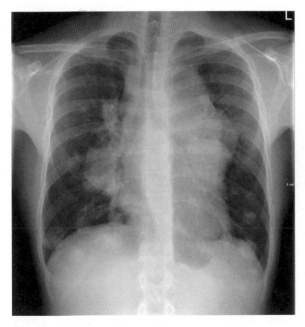

Figure 21.1 Chest radiograph.

Questions

- What abnormalities are seen on the chest radiograph?
- What differential diagnosis would you consider?
- What other investigations would you consider for diagnosis?

ANSWER 21

The chest radiograph shows marked enlargement of the hila and mediastinum with multiple rounded masses. Multiple soft tissue masses are also noted in both lungs. The heart and bones appear normal.

The differential diagnosis to be considered is that of bilateral hilar and mediastinal enlargement with multiple lung masses. The hilar masses are lymph nodes and massively enlarged. The mediastinal masses are likely to be in the anterior or middle mediastinum as the thoracic spine and aortic outlines are clearly seen. At 17, the patient is young enough to consider congenital causes but the recent symptoms and the widespread appearance are suggestive of an acquired disorder. The differential could include neoplastic causes such as lymphoma, leukaemia, germ cell tumour, metastases from sarcoma or possibly a Wilms' tumour, inflammatory lymphadenopathy from tuberculosis, sarcoidosis, histoplasmosis or, less likely, a congenital cause such as lymphatic malformation. The most likely diagnosis is Hodgkin's lymphoma.

Cross-sectional computed tomography (CT) imaging is required (Figure 21.2), also below the diaphragm to assess and stage the extent of disease. A tissue sample is also required and this can be obtained by percutaneous biopsy of an enlarged superficial lymph node (e.g. in the neck) or by endobronchial ultrasound-guided aspiration from a hilar lymph node. Washings can also be taken to rule out tuberculosis.

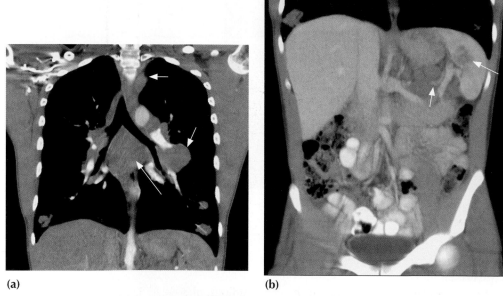

(a)   (b)

Figure 21.2 Coronal computed tomography (CT) slices through (a) the thorax with arrows showing mediastinal, hilar and pulmonary lymphadenopathy; (b) the abdomen showing enlarged pancreatosplenic lymph nodes and a low attenuation lesion in the spleen.

Some nodes have lower attenuation centrally, suggesting necrosis. These finding are significant for the staging and treatment planning. Hodgkin's lymphoma responds well to chemo- and radiotherapy with good long-term survival, and the long-term side effects of treatment must be considered when planning treatment regimes.

The radiology department may be involved in placing an indwelling catheter for regular chemotherapy. Imaging is also required to assess response, typically CT. Subsequently, imaging is used to assess for recurrence and complications.

 KEY POINTS

- On a chest X-ray, mediastinal lymphadenopathy may increase the angle of the carina or give the upper mediastinum a bumpy outline. Increased hilar bulk that does not appear to be vascular may be lymphadenopathy.
- Massive lymphadenopathy is suspicious for lymphoma.

History

A 75-year-old woman is brought into the accident and emergency department following a collapse at home. She has no recollection of the event and appears very confused. Her husband found her on the floor and is worried that she may have hit her head on some furniture. The husband gives a history of his wife being 'under the weather' and 'not quite herself' for several months, although he is unable to explain more specifically. She has otherwise been fit and well and takes medication for blood pressure and for osteoporosis prophylaxis.

Examination

On examination, routine observations are normal. Her Glasgow Coma Score (GCS) is 15 and Mini Mental Test score 6/10. She has mild left-sided limb weakness that appears to be resolving. The chest, cardiovascular and abdominal examination is normal.

You arrange tests including an urgent computed tomography (CT) scan of the head (Figure 22.1), as called for by the National Institute for Health and Clinical Excellence (NICE) guidelines on head injury criteria, including the patient's age and amnesia.

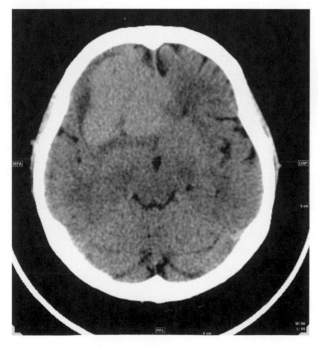

Figure 22.1 Axial non-contrast CT scan through the brain at the level of the quadrigeminal cistern.

Questions

- What does the CT show?
- What would you do next?

The CT shows a large lobulated mass with homogeneously increased attenuation in the right parasagittal frontal lobe. There is mass effect with effacement of the frontal horn of the right lateral ventricle and 1 cm shift of the midline to the left. There is minimal surrounding vasogenic oedema. There is no intracranial haemorrhage or infarct. The basal cisterns are patent.

When considering an intracranial mass, the first step is to decide if the mass arises within the brain (intra-axial), ventricles or cisterns, or from the adjacent structures (extra-axial) such as the meninges or the bone. More imaging using contrast-enhanced magnetic resonance (MR) (or contrast CT if this is not possible) is also done, as this is more sensitive to possible other lesions as well as giving more information about the tumour structure and the surrounding brain (Figure 22.2).

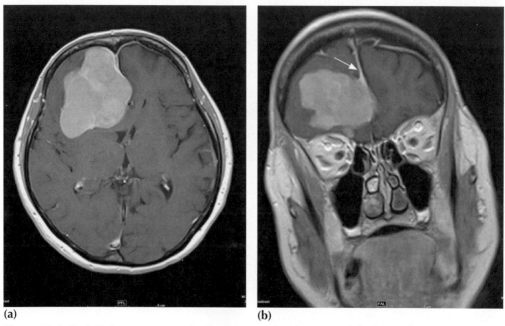

(a) (b)

Figure 22.2 Gadolinium contrast-enhanced T1-weighted images of the brain showing a uniformly enhancing lobulated mass in the right frontal lobe.

The MR shows that the tumour grows from a broad segment of the meninges and appears to be growing along the falx at its edge (see arrow, Figure 22.2b), a so-called dural tail, that is quite characteristic for a meningioma or metastasis (particularly breast). The absence of other lesions and no history of a tumour elsewhere makes a metastasis less likely although it is important to look. Meningiomas frequently have associated calcification and adjacent bone change. The differential also includes intra-axial tumours and lymphoma, although appearance and position make this less likely.

Meningiomas occur intracranially and within the spinal canal arising from the arachnoid layer. They are common, second only to glioblastoma in frequency. The parasagittal position is the most common (33–50 per cent), although other common sites are near the vertex or by the lesser wing of sphenoid or petrous ridge. Ninety per cent are benign but because they grow slowly they can eventually have a space-occupying effect, become symptomatic and as a result tend to be discovered later in life. Surprisingly, the symptoms can seem disproportionately mild for such large tumours. This probably reflects the slow onset and adaptation but also the nature of the prefrontal lobe symptoms, which include change in mentation, apathy or disinhibited behaviour and urinary incontinence that are sometimes attributed to ageing.

 KEY POINTS

- Meningiomas are common, usually benign, relatively silent intracranial tumours.
- The onset and associated symptoms are often insidious and mild until there is a significant mass effect.

Reference

1. National Institute for Health and Clinical Excellence (NICE) (2007) Head injury; triage, assessment, investigation and early management of head injury in infants, children and adults. www.nice.org.uk/nicemedia/live/11836/36257/36257/.pdf

History

A 6-day-old premature baby born at 31 weeks' gestation on the neonatal unit is noted to be lethargic and increasingly intolerant of feeds, with decrease in oxygen saturation and abdominal distension.

Examination

Serial abdominal radiographs are obtained (Figure 23.1 and 23.2).

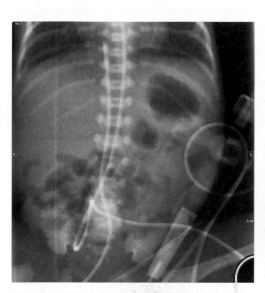

Figure 23.1 Initial radiograph.

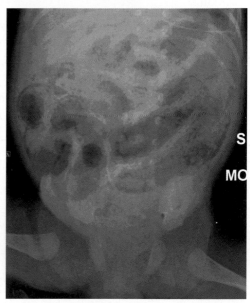

Figure 23.2 Subsequent radiograph.

Questions

- Multiple tubes and lines can be seen in Figure 23.1. What are the two tubes seen in the centre of the radiograph?
- What radiological signs are seen in Figure 23.2?
- What is your differential and most likely diagnosis?

Figure 23.1 shows the abdomen. Two tubes passing over the umbilicus are umbilical artery and vein catheters. They can be distinguished by their course, the umbilical artery catheter passes inferiorly to join the internal iliac artery before passing superiorly. The tip should lie between T6 and T9 vertebral level to avoid major branches. The umbilical venous catheter passes superiorly to the left portal vein, passing through the ductus venosus into the inferior vena cava (IVC). The tip should lie within the upper IVC or at the border with the right atrium. In Figure 23.2, the tip of a nasogastric (NG) tube is seen overlying the stomach. Aspiration and radiographs are typically used to check the position.

The appearances on the first image (Figure 23.1) are non-specific but gas-filled small and large bowel in a symptomatic premature infant should ring alarm bells.

The second image (Figure 23.2) shows dilatation of the bowel (greater than the width of the L1 vertebral body). Bowel wall gas lucencies (pneumatosis intestinalis), particularly in the right lower quadrant and portal venous gas (lucency over the liver) is seen. No evidence of perforation is seen to warrant immediate surgical intervention.

Subsequent images (Figure 23.3) showed further distension and free gas outside the bowel.

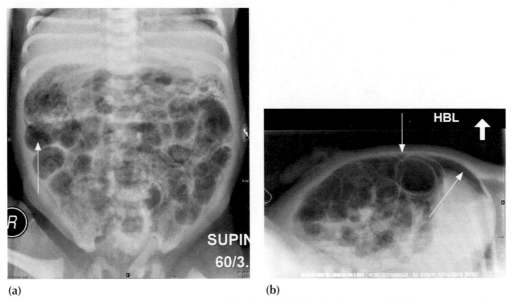

(a)   (b)

Figure 23.3 (a) Anterior–posterior (AP) and (b) lateral abdominal views with the patient supine showing free gas (arrows) above the liver and around the bowel loops, indicating perforation.

The main differential diagnosis is necrotizing enterocolitis and other forms of sepsis. Other differentials include Hirschprung's disease (aganglionic distal colon/rectum), bowel obstruction (such as small bowel atresia, meconium ileus, meconium plug) and ischaemia, particularly in congenital cardiac disease.

Initial management is usually conservative including antibiotics and repeated imaging. Surgery may be required for perforation or failure of medical management.

Necrotizing enterocolitis has a complex aetiology. Immaturity of the gut mucosa and immune response, coupled with ischaemia/hypoxia, are felt to contribute with premature and low birth weight babies at highest risk. Other risk factors more apparent in term infants include sepsis, cyanotic congenital heart disease, polycythaemia and gastroschisis. Long-term complications include strictures and short bowel syndrome.

 KEY POINTS

- A low threshold for suspecting necrotizing enterocolitis in preterm infants is advisable.
- Radiograph findings may be non-specific, although comparing successive images may indicate persistent bowel dilatation, thickening or pneumatosis.
- Management ranges from conservative to surgery if perforation is evident.

History

This 1-year-old girl has been in the paediatric department for a few weeks for treatment of streptococcal sepsis after chickenpox. Around the time of admission the child had swelling over the left upper arm but no abnormality was seen on plain radiograph and there was no collection on ultrasound. After treatment on the paediatric intensive care ward she improved but then started to get intermittent fevers and worsening of the left upper arm swelling.

Examination

The child is irritable and off her feeds. There is tachycardia and pyrexia. Cardiovascular and respiratory examinations are normal. The abdomen is soft and non-tender. Her left arm is not moving, red and swollen over the upper aspect. She complains when you handle or move the arm.

You arrange a plain radiograph and compare it with the previous image (Figure 24.1a,b).

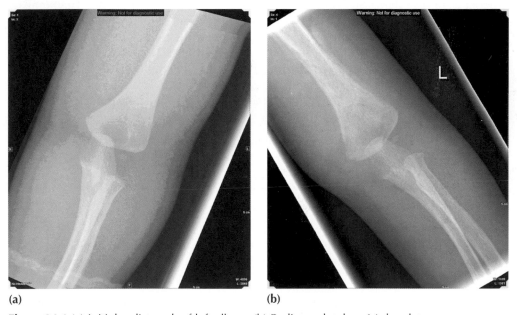

(a)   (b)

Figure 24.1 (a) Initial radiograph of left elbow. (b) Radiograph taken 14 days later.

Questions

• Describe the changes seen.
• What other imaging would you arrange?

The first radiograph (Figure 24.1a) is essentially normal (there may be some soft tissue swelling). The second radiograph (14 days later) (Figure 24.1b) shows thick periosteal reaction along the shaft of the humerus. Patchy lucency is seen within the distal humerus. The appearance is consistent with an aggressive process. Given the acute onset and sepsis, this is likely to be acute osteomyelitis that is an inflammation of bone caused by an infecting organism. The differential for periosteal reaction in an infant could include infiltrative tumour such as leukaemia or neuroblastoma, (non-accidental) trauma, prostaglandin therapy or vitamin deficiency such as rickets (not uncommon) and scurvy (rare).

Osteomyelitis has a bimodal distribution. In children it typically occurs by haematogenous spread with insidious onset. Typical bacteria are *Staphylococcus aureus*, group A *Streptococcus* (in this case), *Haemophilus influenzae* and *Enterobacter* species. Patients with sickle cell disease are particularly at risk of *S. aureus* and *Salmonella* species. The bacteria pass into the metaphysis of the most rapidly growing tubular bones via nutrient vessels where they lodge and cause inflammation, vascular congestion and increased pressure. There may also be some thrombosis. This is followed by a suppurative phase where pus forms subperiosteal abscesses. Increased pressure and thrombosis compromises the blood supply causing bone necrosis and sequestrum formation (fragments of necrotic bone) over a period of days. A layer of new bone, or an involucrum, forms around the raised periosteum. With treatment there is a resolution phase with remodelling of bone. A skin sinus can form in the absence of treatment or as a complication. Other complications in children arise due to damage of the growth plate with deformity or shortening of the developing bone. Haematologically spread osteomyelitis in adults is typically centred in a vertebra.

Direct osteomyelitis is associated with traumatic inoculation, more focal and more typical in adults, particularly those who are at increased risk due to peripheral neuropathy and immune compromise such as diabetic patients. Typical bacteria are *S. aureus*, *Enterobacter* species and *Pseudomonas* species. The development is much the same as described but more focal.

Other imaging that is helpful is a three-phase bone scan that images the whole skeleton and identifies further sites of disease. A magnetic resonance (MR) scan is useful to confirm the diagnosis and examine the soft tissues and bone marrow for abscess formation and complications.

Figure 24.2a,b shows subsequent plain radiographs of the sequestrum phase and resolution.

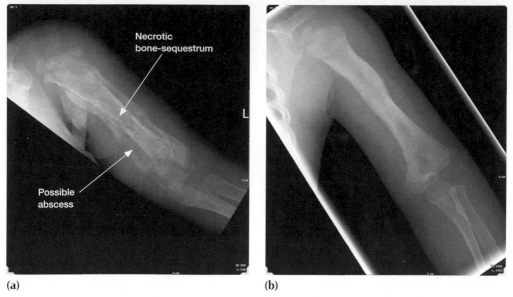

Figure 24.2 Subsequent plain radiographs showing (a) the sequestrum phase and (b) resolution.

🔑 **KEY POINTS**

- Osteomyelitis in children is more commonly caused by haematogenous spread; in adults it is more usually by traumatic inoculation.
- The radiological appearance is aggressive with periosteal reactions and irregular bone resorption, necrosis and reformation.

CASE 25: ACUTE EPIGASTRIC PAIN

History

This 57-year-old woman presented to the accident and emergency department with sudden onset of epigastric pain with vomiting and retching. There is a background history of grumbling epigastric discomfort with loss of appetite and weight but no bowel disturbance. There is no other medical history of note.

Examination

She looks unwell with mild pyrexia and dehydration. The pulse is 96/minute and regular, blood pressure is 122/80 lying and 104/72 standing. The chest examination is otherwise normal. Abdominal examination shows mild distension with no significant scars but it is rigid to palpitation, dull to percussion and very reduced bowel sounds are heard.

Abdominal and erect chest radiographs are obtained (Figure 25.1).

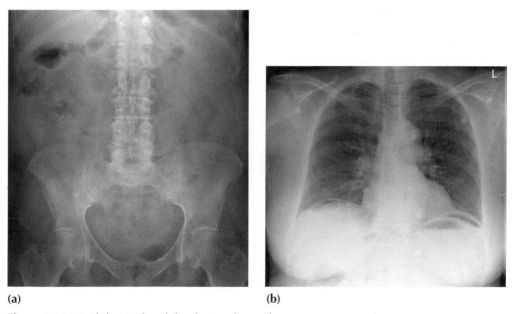

(a)   **(b)**

Figure 25.1 (a) Abdominal and (b) chest radiographs.

Questions

- What abnormality is present on the X-ray?
- What is your differential diagnosis?
- What further imaging would you like to do?

This is a case of acute abdomen. The first priority is to resuscitate and stabilize the patient and as the patient is middle aged and relatively fit, she may be compensating quite well. The abdominal X-ray shows undilated small and large bowel. No classic signs of free gas outside the bowel wall (Rigler's sign), triangular gas pockets or gas outlining the falciform ligament are seen on the abdominal radiograph.

A chest X-ray is part of the investigation of acute abdomen and is obtained after about 5 minutes with the patient sitting as upright as possible. This allows any free intra-abdominal gas to rise, giving the characteristic free gas under the diaphragm sign. This chest radiograph shows free gas below the diaphragm (pneumoperitoneum). Appearances may be deceptive and gas within an organ may look like a perforation. The right upper quadrant is a good place to look as the liver normally abuts the diaphragm and any gas will be obvious. Occasionally the bowel will occupy this space, a condition called Chiladiti's syndrome. Look for characteristic bowel wall folds.

Differential diagnosis for free gas under the diaphragm includes:

- iatrogenic causes – normal appearance after a surgical or laparoscopic procedure or perforation from a surgical anastomosis or after endoscopy;
- perforation due to gastroinstestinal tract disease – gastric/duodenal ulcer, appendix or diverticular perforation, obstruction (e.g. neoplasm) or specific paediatric disorders and inflammatory bowel disease;
- conditions that mimic free gas – pseudopneumoperitoneum, such as distended bowel loops, Chiladiti's syndrome, diaphragmatic hernia, oesophageal diverticulum and sub-phrenic abscess.

A contrast computed tomography (CT) is typically done provided the patient is stable, as the additional anatomical information may help locate the source of perforation (Figure 25.2).

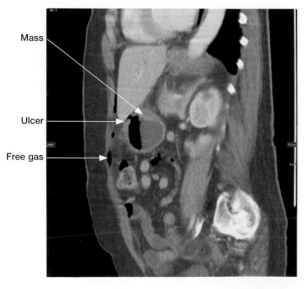

Figure 25.2 Sagittal reconstruction CT slice of the abdomen, showing free gas anterior to the stomach suggesting a perforated gastric ulcer and possible gastric mass. This is useful for the surgeon to know as tissue diagnosis is required and surgical planning may change.

Free gas can be seen after abdominal surgery although a significant quantity of gas 3 days after surgery is suspicious. If available, compare with any previous post-surgical images. CO_2 insufflation used in laparoscopy absorbs rapidly and probably should be gone after 24 hours.

 KEY POINTS

- Plain images of the patient can be done without moving the patient, although to allow free gas to appear under the diaphragm, the patient has to be upright before the chest X-ray.
- There are many causes of pneumoperitoneum and a combination of history and CT may determine the likely cause.

History

A 50-year-old man presented with sudden onset moderate central chest pain. He smokes 15 cigarettes a day and drinks around 10 pints of beer over each weekend. He has had no previous illnesses.

Examination

On examination he looks well. His blood pressure is 164/90 but observations are otherwise normal. Nothing abnormal is found on examination of respiratory, cardiovascular, abdominal and nervous systems. The electrocardiogram (ECG) is normal.

A posterior–anterior (PA) chest radiograph is requested as part of the work up for possible acute coronary syndrome (Figure 26.1).

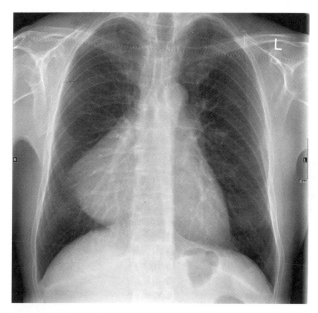

Figure 26.1 PA chest radiograph.

Questions

- What abnormality is present and where is it?
- List some possible differential diagnoses.

The radiograph shows an abnormal but well-defined right heart border. This may reflect cardiac enlargement or a separate soft tissue mass. In general, the position of a soft tissue mass may be indicated by the loss of definition of the edge of adjacent structures – the silhouette sign. In this case the right heart border is abnormal, suggesting a mass adjacent to the right atrium of the heart obscuring the normal air–tissue interface. The differential diagnosis therefore includes anterior and middle mediastinal or lung masses such as pericardial cyst, lipoma, fat pad, bronchogenic cyst, sequestration, massive lymphadenopathy, diaphragmatic hernia, ventricular aneurysm or right atrial enlargement.

A computed tomography (CT) scan is the next step in imaging (Figure 26.2). This not only localizes the abnormality but also displays the soft tissue attenuation (measured in Hounsfield units, HU), which allows distinction between fat (e.g. in a fat pad or lipoma – typically negative HU), water-like fluid (HU <10) in a cyst, soft tissue and contrast (>100 HU) in, for example, a ventricular aneurysm. In this case there is a fluid attenuation mass adjacent to the heart, which otherwise appears normal, consistent with a pericardial cyst. There is also a small area of adjacent right upper lung lobe collapse (atelectasis).

Pericardial cysts are congenital malformations that are attached to the parietal pericardium, but do not communicate with the pericardial space. If there is communication with the pericardial space, the structure is termed a pericardial diverticulum. They are usu-

ally found incidentally in asymptomatic patients. The most frequent location is in the right cardiophrenic angle, but they can be found in the left cardiophrenic angle, anterior mediastinum or middle mediastinum. The vast majority are unilocular and they usually range in size between 3 and 8 cm. Because they are soft, they may change shape with position. Rarely, they may cause symptoms due to compression of surrounding structures and require surgical removal.

Bronchogenic cysts arise out of the tracheobronchial tree as a congenital malformation, typically pericarinal but also paratracheal, oesophageal, retrocardiac and pulmonary in location. They are usually asymptomatic but may cause stridor, compression or become infected.

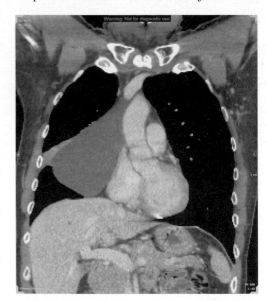

Figure 26.2 Reconstructed coronal CT slice through the thorax.

 KEY POINTS

- Pericardial cysts are occasionally incidental, asymptomatic findings on chest X-ray.
- They abut the heart, resulting in a silhouette sign, and may be diagnosed on CT if they have classic cystic appearance.

History

This 37-year-old woman presents to the accident and emergency department after referral from her general practitioner (GP) complaining of increasing breathlessness and intermittent right-sided chest pain. The symptoms have come on over 2–3 weeks without associated fever or significant cough. There is a medical history of pelvic pain that is undergoing investigation for suspected endometriosis. She is otherwise well, a non-smoker and taking no medication.

Examination

The right hemithorax is dull to percussion with reduced breath sounds throughout. The left lung and heart sound normal. The abdomen is soft and there is tenderness to palpation diffusely over both iliac fossae.

You arrange some tests including a chest radiograph (Figure 27.1).

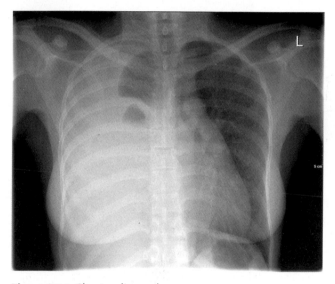

Figure 27.1 Chest radiograph.

Questions

- What is the main abnormality and what effect is it having on the normal anatomy?
- What is the differential diagnosis?
- What is the appropriate management?

ANSWER 27

There is uniform opacification of most of the right hemithorax. The right hemidiaphragm and heart border are not seen. There is displacement of the heart and trachea to the left. Some residual aerated right lung is noted, probably the apices of the right upper and lower lobes. The left lung and heart are normal in appearance. No bone abnormality is seen.

We are looking for causes of opacification of a hemithorax. This can be within the lung, mediastinum or pleural space and may involve consolidation, soft tissue or fluid. The position of the mediastinum gives a clue as it is displaced away from the opacity even though the lung only appears partially aerated. This suggests a differential of pleural fluid or soft tissue, such as from a diaphragmatic hernia. Other causes such as consolidation, lung collapse, tumours (such as mesothelioma) or congenital agenesis or hypoplasia tend either not to displace or to displace the mediastinum towards the opacity. The appearance with smooth edges and some thickening of the horizontal fissure suggests pleural effusion.

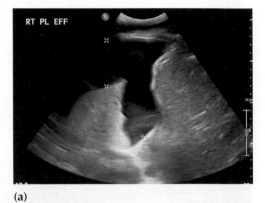

Effusions can be transudates (protein <30 g/L; e.g. in cardiac failure), exudates (>30 g/L; e.g. in infection, malignancy, pulmonary infarction), haemorrhagic (e.g. trauma, carcinoma) or chylous (e.g. due to obstructed thoracic duct caused by trauma, malignancy or parasites). Systemic diseases often cause bilateral effusions but can be unilateral.

(a)

To investigate this further, cross-sectional imaging to determine the underlying cause may be done. Computed tomography (CT) is not typically sensitive to the type of effusion. The effusion may also be drained, particularly if the patient is symptomatic, and a sample of fluid may help to decide on the cause. This is typically done with ultrasound guidance (Figure 27.2a), often using a Seldinger technique with a needle to insert a guidewire over which a drain tube is inserted. Thoracoscopy may be performed to look into the pleural space and allows biopsy of any abnormal pleural tissue. Figure 27.2b shows the result of drainage. The effusion in this case was stained with old blood and eventually shown to be caused by an endometriosis deposit.

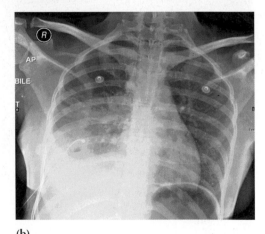

(b)

Figure 27.2 (a) Ultrasound of the right lung base; (b) anterior–posterior (AP) radiograph showing a right basal chest drain and partial drainage of the effusion.

 KEY POINTS

- There are multiple causes of thoracic opacification and noting the effect on the mediastinum and anatomy helps to narrow down the possible causes.
- Consider pleural effusions in terms of transudate, exudates, blood and chyle.

History

A 68-year-old man on treatment for non-Hodgkin's lymphoma presents to the accident and emergency department with mild chest discomfort, worse on lying flat and eased by leaning forward. It has been getting slowly worse over the last few weeks. Now he gets dizzy on standing, rapidly breathless on exertion and has noticed some bilateral ankle swelling over the last week. He does not have a significant past cardiac or respiratory history.

Examination

On examination his blood pressure is 144/88, pulse 94/minute and respiratory rate 22/minute. The JVP is a little raised and fine crackles are heard at both lung bases. The heart sounds are difficult to hear but otherwise regular. The abdomen is soft and there is moderate left flank tenderness to deep palpation. The electrocardiogram (ECG) shows small QRS complexes and T wave inversion.

You organize a chest radiograph as well as blood tests (Figure 28.1).

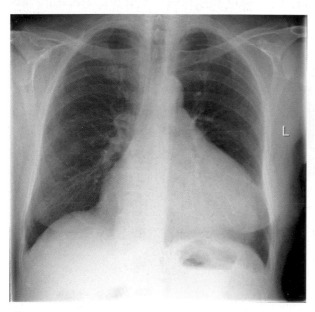

Figure 28.1 Posterior–anterior (PA) chest radiograph.

Questions

- What abnormalities are seen?
- What others symptoms or signs might you find?
- What other tests would you do?

The heart is enlarged. The hilar vessels are not enlarged. There is some blunting of the costophrenic angles but no lung abnormality is seen.

The heart size is usually estimated by measuring the cardiothoracic ratio (CTR, maximum cardiac width/maximum inner thoracic width) on a PA projection radiograph with adequate inspiration (6 ribs seen anteriorly, 10 posteriorly). Beware anterior–posterior (AP) projections and poor inspiration as this will artificially increase the size of the heart. Typically in adults a CTR ratio >0.5 suggests cardiomegaly.

In addition to the CTR, the heart shape may indicate an underlying cause such as valve disease or a shunt. Increase of the right atrium size shifts the right heart border laterally; the left ventricle shifts the left heart border. The right ventricle lifts the heart, moving the apex superolaterally. The left atrium is behind the heart and on enlarging may project a second border over the right side of the heart. The left atrial appendage may enlarge and may produce a bump at the upper left heart border. Often the heart just appears generally enlarged and correlates with heart failure; occasionally this may be due to a pericardial effusion and is termed the 'water bottle sign'.

The differential diagnosis for cardiomegaly includes ischaemic heart disease, valve disease, pericardial effusion/cardiac tamponade, dilated cardiomyopathy and pulmonary embolism. In this patient, the presentation is suspicious for a pericardial effusion, probably malignant in origin and is confirmed on computed tomography (CT) (Figure 28.2).

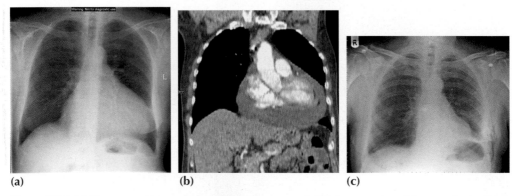

(a) (b) (c)

Figure 28.2 (a) The presenting radiograph, (b) the coronal CT shows a rim of lower attenuation fluid around the heart, (c) radiograph after paracentesis.

The pericardium covers the heart and great vessels, with the exception of only partially covering the left atrium and normally contains less than 50 mL of transudate fluid. To be distinctive on chest X-ray more than 250 mL needs to be present. The type of excess fluid depends on the cause:

- transudate – congestive heart failure, hypoalbuminaemia;
- exudate – infection, autoimmune disease (e.g. rheumatoid arthritis, systemic lupus erythematosus, hypersensitivity);
- blood – trauma, surgery, rupture, myocardial infarction, neoplasm;
- lymph – neoplasm, surgery.

An echocardiogram is the next investigation of choice and may be used to guide insertion of a pericardial drain.

KEY POINTS

- A cardiothoracic ratio greater than 0.5 on a PA projection radiograph with good inspiration indicates cardiomegaly.
- Pericardial effusions are difficult to see on chest X-ray unless large, although a rapid change in heart size on successive X-rays is suspicious.

History

A 13-year-old boy was skateboarding when he fell forwards onto steps and twisted his right foot. His description of the injury sounds as if it involved inversion of the foot. He is taking no medication and there is no significant medical history.

Examination

The boy is a fit 13 year old who appears well but in discomfort. The right mid foot is swollen and tender, more over the lateral aspect. The ankle joint is not painful but there is pain in the foot on moving the ankle joint. There are no other injuries.

You arrange plain radiographs of the right foot (Figure 29.1).

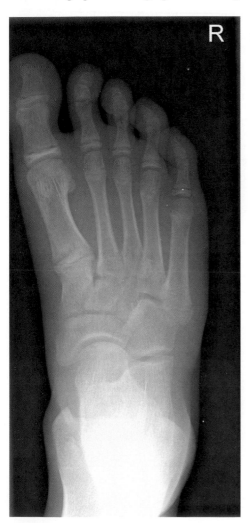

Figure 29.1 Anterior–posterior radiograph of the right foot.

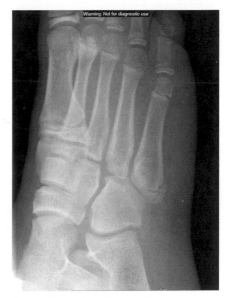

Figure 29.2 Magnified oblique radiograph of the right foot.

Questions

- Given the history, where would you look for an injury?
- What do the radiographs show?
- What might be confusing about the appearance of this injury?
- What other foot fractures should you consider?

ANSWER 29

Given the history of inversion, a common injury, the lateral side of the foot, particularly the base of the fifth metatarsal should be checked. Forced dorsiflexion suggests the shafts of the metatarsal and phalanges could also be injured.

The radiographs show a complex lucency through the base of the right fifth metatarsal, in keeping with a fracture (Figure 29.2). There is associated soft tissue swelling. No other fractures are seen.

The appearance of the fracture is complex. Reviewing the whole foot, multiple epiphyses are noted consistent with a 13 year old with active growth plates which may cause some confusion in interpretation of the radiographs. An unfused apophysis (secondary ossification centre) lies parallel to the lateral edge of the base of the fifth metatarsal. The transverse fracture line crosses the apophysis and base of the metatarsal. Fractures at the base of the fifth metatarsal are common and reflect an avulsion injury of the peroneus brevis tendon, typically on inverting the foot. The fracture edge is typically at right angles to the metatarsal lateral cortex and should not be confused with the apophysis, if present. There may also be an ossicle close the fifth metatarsal base. Ossicles should have a smooth outline with a regular or corticated edge.

Other common foot injuries to be considered that can be subtle in appearance are:

- Lisfranc fractures (see Case 87), in which the Lisfranc ligament at the base of the first to fourth metatarsals is injured; there may be avulsion fragments between the first and second metatarsal bases and the alignment of the metatarsal shafts and cuneiforms is lost;
- avulsions, appearing as small flakes of bone around the interphalangeal joints where the flexor, extensor tendons insert;
- stress fractures of the shafts of predominantly second and third metatarsals in long distance runners or people with a walking injury; these may be difficult to see and appear initially only as a periosteal reaction;
- fracture through the first metatarsal ossicles.

KEY POINTS

- The mechanism of injury and site of symptoms may help to find subtle injuries.
- It is important to look around the edge of every bone, as small avulsions and stress fracture periosteal reactions are easy to miss.
- Review the whole foot and beware of 'satisfaction of search' – where you stop looking after finding an injury. Multiple injuries are common in trauma.

History

A 24-year-old man presents with sudden onset left upper quadrant pain radiating to the groin with mild haematuria. He has no history of previous episodes or past renal problems. There is no history of lower urinary tract symptoms. He is otherwise fit and well with no medical problems or relevant family history. He smokes 10 cigarettes per day and drinks around 10 units of alcohol per week.

Examination

He is well with a pulse of 94 per minute but otherwise normal observations. The chest examination is normal with normal heart sounds. The abdomen is soft but tender on the left side, most notably over the left renal angle and left inguinal fossa. Urinalysis shows blood 4+ but no protein or nitrites.

You arrange an urgent intravenous urogram (IVU) (Figure 30.1).

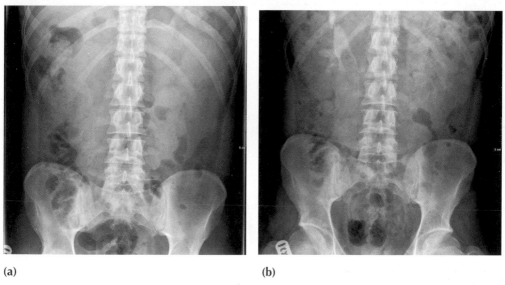

(a)   (b)

Figure 30.1 (a) Control and (b) 20-minute images from an intravenous urogram. Pelvic views were normal.

Questions

• What is a urogram?
• What are you looking for on the control image and do you see any abnormality?
• What does the 20-minute image show?
• What is the differential diagnosis?

An IVU consists of a control image without contrast to look for calcification. Contrast is then given intravenously and images are taken while the contrast passes through the kidneys (nephrogram phase) and then as it drains through the collecting system and ureters into the bladder. The IVU is becoming a rather old-fashioned test because it provides only limited anatomical information and is being replaced by pre, post and delayed contrast phase computed tomography (CT).

The control image (Figure 30.2a) is reviewed for calculi (none seen) and the renal outline, which in this case appears enlarged and lobulated bilaterally (Figure 30.2b).

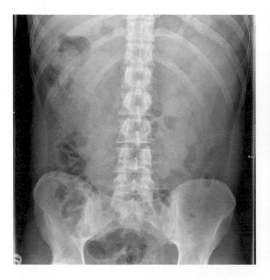 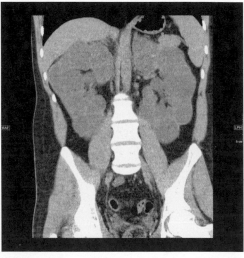

(b)

Figure 30.2 (a) Control and (b) corresponding coronal CT slice demonstrating the renal outline and appearance.

The 20-minute IVU radiograph shows drainage of contrast through the collecting system on the right that has a slightly distorted appearance. No drainage is seen on the left, suggesting obstruction, confirmed on later images with a delayed nephrogram and slow accumulation of contrast in a dilated collecting system and due to a small stone, not seen on the plain images, at about the level of the pelviureteric junction (outflow of the left kidney) seen on CT.

There is an underlying bilateral kidney disorder with lobulated increase in size due to cyst formation. The differential for cystic diseases of the kidney includes acquired simple cysts (most common with increasing age and few in number), developmental disorders (e.g. multicystic dysplastic kidney), genetic causes (e.g. autosomal recessive (ARPKD) and dominant (ADPKD) polycystic kidney disease), systemic diseases (e.g. Von Hippel–Lindau syndrome and tuberous sclerosis) or malignancy in the form of cystic renal cell carcinoma. This patient has newly diagnosed ADPKD.

Unlike ARPKD that presents in childhood with renal failure and may be diagnosed prenatally, ADPKD is often clinically silent until it presents in adulthood, either with complications such as stones, haematuria, hypertension or renal failure (typically mean age for endstage renal failure is over 50). However, as an autosomal dominant disease, the patient may be aware of a family history of renal disease and may present for ultrasound screening. Cysts may be seen in other organs and there is an association with cardiac and vascular anomalies, such as intracranial berry aneurysms.

 KEY POINTS

- There are many causes of renal cysts; sporadic simple cysts are the most common.
- ADPKD typically becomes symptomatic later in life and is a significant cause of endstage renal failure.

History

A 45-year-old woman presents to the accident and emergency department after collision with a car while on her bicycle. She complains that the car hit her left knee from the side and she is unable to bend the knee or support her weight. Previously she was fit and well.

Examination

She is initially immobilized with a hard collar. Her neck, chest and abdomen examination is unremarkable and plain images of the neck, chest and pelvis are normal. The left knee appears swollen and bruised but there is no penetrating injury. Plain anterior–posterior (AP) and lateral radiographs of the knee are taken (Figure 31.1a,b).

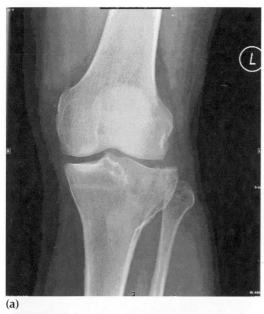

(a)

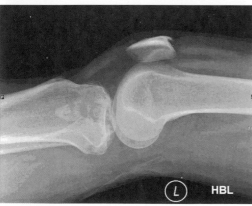

Figure 31.1 (a) AP and (b) lateral radiographs of the left knee.

Questions

- What abnormality is seen?
- What would you do next?

There is a horizontal fat–fluid line, a lipohaemarthrosis, in the suprapatella pouch seen on the cross-table horizontal lateral view. There is also a fracture of the lateral tibial plateau, seen on the AP projection, with minimal displacement and loss of height.

A lipohaemarthrosis results from an intra-articular fracture with escape of fat and blood from the bone marrow into the joint. Ideally the patient has been lying supine for 5 minutes to allow the fat and blood to separate. The fat rises and is less radio-opaque. If seen, a lipohaemarthrosis indicates a tibial plateau or distal femoral fracture even if the fracture is not apparent. Conversely, in a significant proportion of tibial fractures a lipohaemarthrosis is not seen, although a haemarthrosis or effusion that appears as soft tissue without a fluid level in the suprapatella bursa is likely to be present.

A computed tomography (CT) scan is done to image the extent of injury and plan surgery (Figure 31.2).

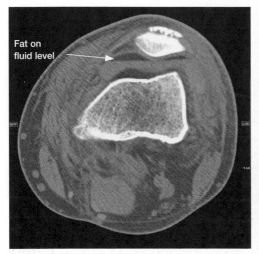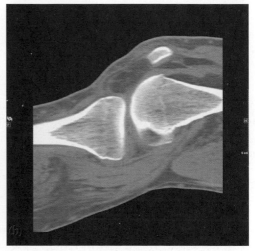

Figure 31.2 (a) Axial and (b) sagittal CT slices of the right knee demonstrating the suprapatellar lipohaemarthrosis.

There are a number of classification systems, such as the Schatzker classification, that recognize patterns of fragmentation and displacement for tibial fractures. It is important to recognize that a significant proportion of fractures will have associated meniscal, collateral and cruciate ligamentous injury. These are better assessed by magnetic resonance (MR) which can also identify occult fractures.

Tibial plateau fractures may be either low or high energy. The majority of tibial plateau fractures are in patients over 50 years. Osteoporosis in older women is a contributing factor in low energy fractures and typically results in a depressed fracture. Tibial plateau fractures in younger patients are commonly the result of high energy injuries. The most common mechanism is a valgus force at the knee while weight bearing or with axial loading, typically either road traffic accidents or sports-related injuries.

 KEY POINTS

- A fat–fluid level in the suprapatella bursa indicates a lipohaemarthrosis and is likely to indicate a tibial plateau fracture even if not seen on plain radiographs.
- Increased size of the suprapatella bursa most likely indicates an effusion or a haemarthrosis.

History

A 77-year-old woman presents to the accident and emergency department after slipping on ice and falling, hurting her left hip. She is unable to weight bear on her left leg. There is no history of significant past joint pain or swelling. Before falling she had mildly limited mobility but was otherwise active and well. Other than bendroflumethiazide for hypertension there is no significant medical history.

Examination

The left leg is shortened with deformity around the hip. There is bruising over the lateral aspect but no neurological or vascular abnormality is noted in the leg. Her observations and the rest of the examination are normal.

You organize a pelvic and left hip radiograph and review a previous image of the left hip (Figure 32.1).

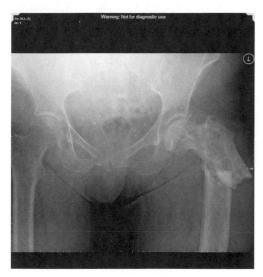
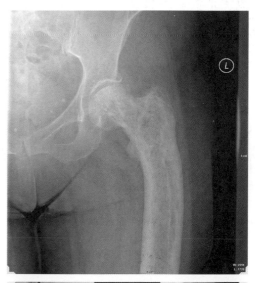
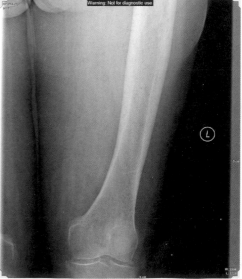

Figure 32.1 Current AP pelvic radiographs (left) and AP hip radiograph (right) from 1 year earlier.

Questions

- What abnormality is seen on the pelvic radiograph.
- What is the differential diagnosis for this appearance?
- What would you do next?

The pelvic radiograph shows a fracture through the proximal femoral shaft with displacement of the distal femur and angulation of the proximal fragment. The radiographs also show a longstanding abnormal bony appearance of most of the left femur with expansion (compared with the right), cortical thickening and trabecular coarsening, most prominent around the femoral head and neck. There is also bowing of the femoral shaft.

The differential diagnosis includes Paget's disease, osteomyelitis, metastatic carcinoma and myelofibrosis. Trabecular coarsening and cortical thickening is quite characteristic of Paget's disease. There is no history or other findings to suggest metastatic cancer (typically multiple sclerotic lesions in breast or prostatic cancer) or osteomyelitis, and the asymmetry makes myelofibrosis less likely.

Paget's disease is a disorder of bone remodelling which may occur in single or multiple bones and typically affects spine, pelvis, femur and skull. The aetiology is not known, however, the disease progresses through a resorption, lytic phase with excessive osteoclastic activity to a bone formation osteoblastic sclerotic phase with a mixed phase in between. Paget's disease occurs predominantly in older patients, affecting less than 3 per cent of patients around 50, rising to as much as 10 per cent in the over 80s. There is a slightly higher incidence in Europeans and males.

Figure 32.2 demonstrates Paget's disease in other bones. In the spine, the vertebral bodies typically become enlarged with a prominent cortical margin (picture frame vertebrae) or become sclerotic, mimicking lymphoma or metastatic disease. In the pelvis, typical findings include thickening of the iliopectineal line (see arrows, Figure 32.2a) in early stages, progressing to patchy sclerosis and lucency in later stages.

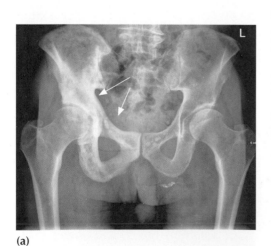 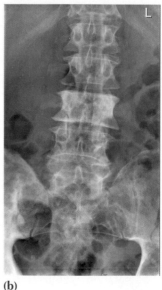

(a)   (b)

Figure 32.2 Paget's disease in (a) the right side of the pelvis and (b) an L3 vertebral body of different patients.

Complications of Paget disease depend on the bone and stage of disease. The majority of people with Paget's disease are asymptomatic, but those with symptoms may experience bone pain (most common symptom), osteoarthritis of adjacent joints, insufficiency fractures, bowing of affected long bones, excessive warmth (due to hypervascularity) and neurologic complications such as deafness and cranial nerve involvement, particularly when the spine or skull is involved. Beware of sarcomatous change in 1 per cent of patients (rising to 5–10 per cent if more than one bone is affected).

 KEY POINTS

- Paget's disease is usually asymptomatic and a not infrequent incidental finding in older people.
- The disease typically affects spine, pelvis, femur and skull, and characteristically demonstrates cortical thickening, trabecular coarsening late in the disease, although lucency is a feature of early Paget's disease.

History
A 15-year-old girl presents to the accident and emergency department with lower back pain following a fall while taking part in gymnastics at school. She complains of a history of lower back discomfort. There is otherwise no significant medical history.

Examination
She is in pain but otherwise well. There is diffuse tenderness over the lower lumbar vertebrae but no point tenderness to suggest a fracture.

Anterior–posterior and lateral lumbar spine X-rays are obtained (Figure 33.1).

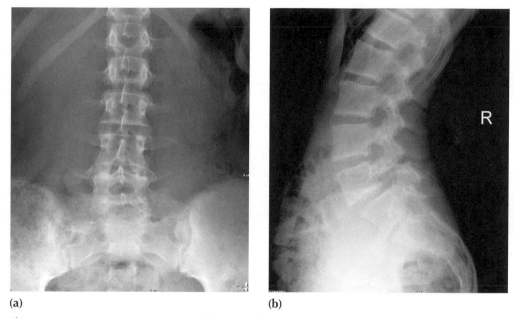

(a)   **(b)**

Figure 33.1 (a) Anterior–posterior and (b) lateral lumbar spine radiographs.

Questions
- What do the plain images show?
- Which part of the anatomy is affected?
- What other imaging would be helpful?

ANSWER 33

The lateral image demonstrates anterior slip of L5 on S1 by about 25 per cent of the vertebral width, otherwise termed spondylolisthesis or anterolisthesis. The degree of slip is graded in steps of 25 per cent (i.e. <25 per cent grade 1, 25–50 per cent grade 2, etc.). A lucency is seen through the pars interarticularis – the portion of the neural arch that connects the superior and inferior articular facets, suggesting a bony defect. This is otherwise known as spondylolysis. On oblique radiographs, the posterior elements form the appearance of a Scottie dog and a break in the pars interarticularis has the appearance of a collar around the neck.

A computed tomography (CT) scan has been obtained to examine the bony structures (Figure 33.2). Magnetic resonance (MR) would be useful if the nerve roots or spinal cord need to be imaged, although the bony structures are less well seen.

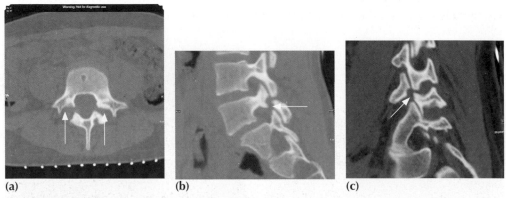

(a)　　　　　　　　　　　(b)　　　　　　　　　　　(c)

Figure 33.2 (a) Axial, (b) sagittal and (c) oblique CT slices through the L5 vertebra showing bilateral pars defects (see arrows), widening of the spinal canal and a 'Scottie dog' projection with the pars defect representing the dog's collar.

Spondylolysis is thought to be caused by stress fracturing of the pars from repeated minor trauma and may occur early in life. Hereditary pars hypoplasia is also believed to be a factor. Patients with spina bifida occulta have an increased risk for spondylolysis. Spondylolysis can also occur secondary to neoplasm, osteomalacia, osteomyelitis and bone disorders such as Paget's disease and osteogenesis imperfecta.

The L5 vertebra is most frequently affected, a smaller proportion at L4 or L3, and it is unusual for spondylolysis to occur at several levels. Seventy-five per cent are bilateral. Lyses occur much less commonly at other lumbar or the thoracic levels.

Patients with bilateral pars defects can develop spondylolisthesis. The vertebral body slips forward while the posterior elements remain fixed so that the spinal canal widens. Stability is provided by the soft tissues and ligaments. Degenerative change is a more common cause in older patients. Increased motion of the facet joints allows movement but slip of the intact vertebra results in spinal canal stenosis and symptoms. Treatment depends on the type of slip, age of patient and symptoms and ranges from conservative management to surgical fixation.

 KEY POINTS

- Spondylolysis is a defect through the pars interarticularis, usually at L5 or L4, probably the result of stress fracturing.
- Spondylolisthesis is slip, usually anteriorly, of one vertebral body on another and may be the result of spondylolysis in younger patients or, more commonly, degenerative change in older patients.

History

A 6-week-old boy is referred urgently to the paediatric department by his general practitioner (GP) with a 1-week history of vomiting after feeds and weight loss. His mother
describes forceful vomiting occurring during or shortly after feeds; the vomit does not
appear bile stained. He appears to have normal appetite and no other symptoms. No other
members of the family seem affected.

Examination

The baby is apyrexial, mildly dehydrated with normal observations. The chest is clear and
abdomen soft and not distended. There is a small palpable mass in the right upper quadrant and after feeding some peristalsis under the skin in the epigastic region is observable.
You organize an ultrasound scan of the upper abdomen (Figure 34.1).

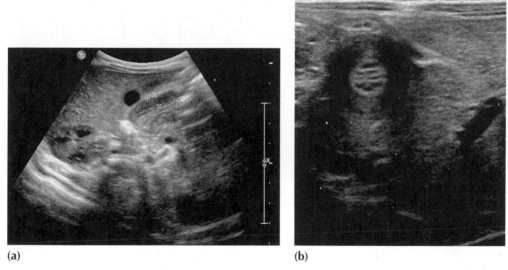

(a)   (b)

Figure 34.1 (a) Transverse and (b) longitudinal ultrasound images through the liver and adjacent
structures.

Questions

- Which organs lie immediately behind the liver?
- What is the differential and most likely diagnosis?
- Are there any risk factors?
- What is the treatment?

Figure 34.1a shows a transverse ultrasound view of the right upper quadrant with a prominent tubular pylorus just behind the liver in keeping with pyloric stenosis. By viewing the pylorus over a period of time (if baby allows), altered pyloric function can be viewed with limited or absent flow of stomach contents through to the duodenum and ineffective gastric peristalsis, which may sometimes be observable by eye. Pyloric muscle thicker than 4 mm, length >17 mm and transverse diameter >14 mm are criteria sometimes used, although this will depend on the age of the baby. Figure 34.2 shows transverse ultrasound with measurements.

Pyloric stenosis is the most common cause of intestinal obstruction in infancy (2–4 per 1000). It is due to hypertrophy and hyperplasia of the muscular layers with thickening and lengthening of the pylorus, causing functional gastric outlet obstruction. Typical features are presentation at 2–8 weeks (although can present up to 5 months). The pylorus may be palpable, about the size of a large olive. Forceful, projectile vomiting that is not bile stained is suggestive of pyloric obstruction. Blood tests typically indicate hypochloraemic alkalosis, due to vomiting gastric acid, and dehydration.

The differential diagnosis includes:

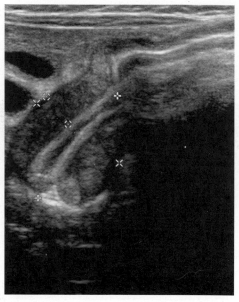

Figure 34.2 Transverse ultrasound with measurements. The gastric mucosa is bright, the muscle dark.

- infections including gastroenteritis and urinary tract;
- gastritis, gastroesophageal reflux, hiatus hernia;
- malrotation, pyloric atresia, web or diaphragm;
- congenital adrenal hyperplasia (due to metabolic imbalance);
- poor feeding practices.

If the diagnosis is not clear on ultrasound, a contrast meal and follow through that examines the stomach and small bowel is the next step. Pyloric stenosis typically shows shouldering of the gastric antrum outlet with a long, narrow pyloric canal (string sign) on a contrast meal. Malrotation and other causes of outflow obstruction also show characteristic appearances.

There is a higher incidence of pyloric stenosis in first-born boys (M:F 4:1). There is also evidence for heritability and that the condition appears to be developmental rather than congenital. The definitive treatment is surgical pyloromyotomy, where the pylorus muscle is cut longitudinally to release the pyloric tension.

 KEY POINTS

- Pyloric stenosis typically presents within 2–12 weeks as non-bilious vomiting.
- Ultrasound appearances can be diagnostic with the pylorus appearing lengthened and thickened and no significant flow of stomach contents through to the duodenum.

History

A 68-year-old woman is referred to the radiology department for an urgent chest radiograph after an abnormality is noted in the left kidney on ultrasound in the urology clinic. She has a recent history of painless haematuria.

Examination

There is little of note on general examination except that she looks thin. There is mild diffuse tenderness in the right loin and a possible ballotable mass on the right.

You review the chest radiograph (Figure 35.1) before the patient leaves the department.

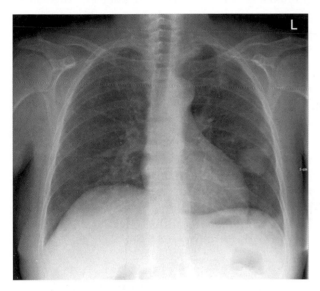

Figure 35.1 Posterior–anterior (PA) chest radiograph.

Questions

- What does the radiograph show?
- What is the differential for this appearance?
- What imaging would you do next?

ANSWER 35

The chest radiograph shows several circular soft tissue lesions in both hemithoraces, most prominent on the left.

The first issue is how to describe the lesions. Convention is that a 'nodule' is smaller and a 'mass' larger than 3 cm. Nodules can be thought of as miliary (multiple, with size and appearance of seeds), small (2–5 mm) or large (>5 mm). They may be single or multiple, discrete or confluent, uniform or variable in size, contain calcification or cavities and be associated with lymphadenopathy, pleural effusions or pleural or rib lesions. Noting these features can help to narrow down the list of differentials.

In this case the list of differentials for multiple variable size soft tissue pulmonary nodules includes metastases, Wegener's granulomatosis, rheumatoid nodules, sarcoidosis, amyloidosis (often calcified), arteriovenous malformations and abscesses. Most likely are metastases from a possible renal primary. Metastases often have a rounded mass appearance, having grown rapidly from a bloodborne deposit, whereas primary lung tumours often have an irregular, infiltrative or spiculated appearance.

The lungs are one of the most common sites for haematogenous spread of tumours, particularly from kidney, osteosarcoma, thyroid, melanoma and breast. When that list is adjusted for tumour incidence, lung metastases are most commonly seen for breast, kidney, head and neck, and colorectal tumours.

A computed tomography (CT) scan to characterize the kidney lesion and to stage the disease is required (Figure 35.2). In particular, evidence of any growth of the tumour into surrounding structures or lymph nodes or into the renal vein or opposite kidney will alter the treatment. Renal tumours account for 3 per cent of adult tumours and the large majority are renal cell carcinomas (RCCs). Thirty per cent of patients with RCC present with metastases, which in addition to lung occur in soft tissue, bone and liver.

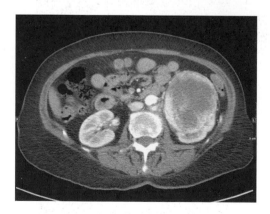

Figure 35.2 Axial contrast-enhanced CT through the kidneys showing a large left renal tumour.

 KEY POINTS

- The size, number, distribution and properties of lung nodules can help decide the differential diagnosis.
- Kidney, osteosarcoma, thyroid, melanoma and breast tumours most commonly metastasize to the lungs.
- Renal cell carcinoma is the most common adult kidney cancer.

History

An 80-year-old woman was brought into the accident and emergency department from her sheltered accommodation with sudden onset right-sided weakness and slurred speech. She is not known to have had a previous stroke or neurological symptoms. She has a past history of chronic obstructuve pulmonary disease (COPD) and 50 pack-years smoking.

Examination

There is right-sided leg and arm weakness (3/5), mild slurring of speech and left facial droop. The chest is clear and abdomen soft and non-tender. Observations show a regular heart rate of 72/minute, blood pressure of 132/82 and no pyrexia. A computed tomography (CT) scan of the head is arranged (Figure 36.1).

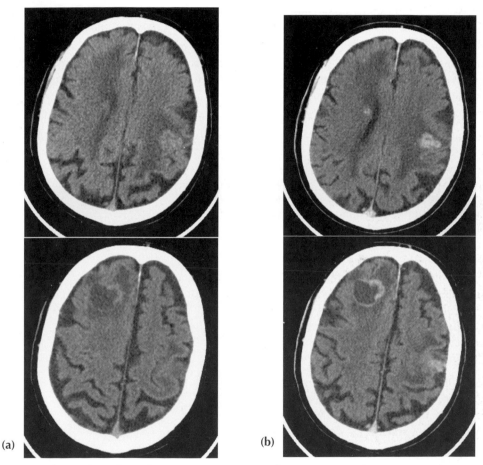

(a)　　　　(b)

Figure 36.1 Axial CT slices through brain at two levels: (a) images without contrast; (b) images with contrast.

Questions

- What is the differential diagnosis for 'stroke'?
- What does the CT demonstrate?
- Is contrast used regularly for head CTs?
- What is your most likely diagnosis and what other investigations would you arrange?

ANSWER 36

The aim of imaging is early diagnosis and to differentiate ischaemic and haemorrhagic stroke. Stroke mimics include space-occupying lesions such as tumours, haematomas, arterial dissections, abscess and acute infection (often a urinary tract infection) in patients with chronic cerebral degeneration such as dementia.

The computed tomography (CT) shows low attenuation regions within the subcortical white matter of the superior right frontal lobe and posterior left frontal lobe in the region of the motor cortex. A small central high attenuation area is in keeping with haemorrhage with surrounding white matter oedema. Post contrast, both regions show avid ring enhancement.

Head CTs are almost always initially non-contrast. This is primarily to avoid obscuring acute haemorrhage or haematoma that has mildly increased attenuation compared with the surrounding brain. It also allows calcification to be identified. There are a number of locations where calcification accumulates physiologically, including the choroid plexi (posterior horns of the lateral ventricles), pineal gland and habenula (posterior end of the third ventricle), falx, basal ganglia and vascular atheroma. Physiological calcification is often symmetrically arranged or on the midline. Other calcifications may arise in lesions associated with tumours (e.g. meningiomas), infection, arteriovenous malformations or aneurysms, old haemorrhage and past surgery.

Contrast is given to improve the visibility of the vasculature (e.g. aneurysm, arterovenous malformation) or lesions that often have abnormal vessels with defective blood–brain barrier so that contrast is retained in the tissue.

The ring-enhancing lesions in this patient's case are most likely to be metastatic tumour deposits from a remote primary. A primary brain tumour is less likely in this age group and the clinical picture is not typical for brain abscesses, although the appearance would be quite similar. A chest radiograph would be the next investigation (Figure 36.2), given the history of smoking, although a staging CT of the chest, abdomen and pelvis would be required for treatment planning.

Only a few tumours account for about 95 per cent of brain metastases, most commonly bronchial carcinoma, breast, gastrointestinal tract, renal cell carcinoma and melanoma.

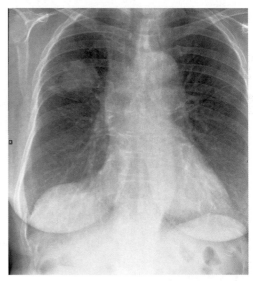

Figure 36.2 Chest radiograph showing a right mid zone mass and hilar lymphadenopathy.

 KEY POINTS

- Although infarction is the most common cause of stroke symptoms, if the patient is young or the history is inconsistent, consider stroke mimics such as tumours or arterial dissections.
- Bronchial cancer is the most common metastasis to the brain.

CASE 37: YOUNG MAN WITH ANKLE PAIN

History

A 20-year-old man presents to the accident and emergency department with a painful right ankle after twisting during football practice. He is barely able to put his weight on the foot. The description sounds like an eversion injury. There is no other or previous injury and the patient is otherwise fit and well. There is no significant medical history.

Examination

On examination the patient appears fit and well but in pain. There is swelling and tenderness over the right lateral malleolus. There is reduced range of movement at the ankle joint. Observations are normal and there are no other significant findings.

You arrange radiographs of the ankle (Figure 37.1).

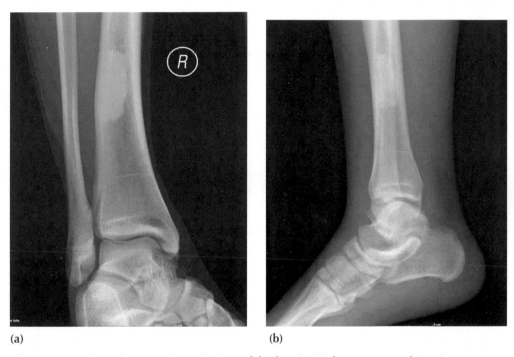

(a) (b)

Figure 37.1 (a) Anterior–posterior (AP) view of the foot in 20 degrees external rotation to see the ankle mortice with minimum overlap; (b) lateral view of the ankle.

Questions

- What do the radiographs show?
- How would you describe the abnormality?
- What are the features that help with a differential diagnosis?
- What are your most likely differentials?

The radiographs show a well-defined sclerotic lesion that is eccentrically positioned in the distal femoral diaphysis. It appears to arise from the cortex and there is no associated bony expansion, soft tissue swelling or periosteal reaction. The ankle joint is normally positioned and regular in appearance. No fracture is seen. There is soft tissue swelling over the lateral malleolus.

When reviewing the ankle it is important to check the joint space between the talus and tibia/fibula which should be the same throughout. Small irregularities within the joint space might indicate an osteochondral defect. Check for avulsion below the fibula and posterior to the fifth metatarsal. Take care not to confuse fractures with ossicles commonly in this position and also posterior to the tibia.

There is quite a structured way of describing bony abnormalities that helps with deriving a differential diagnosis. Consider:

- age;
- number of lesions (may require more imaging);
- location;
- position within the bone (i.e. diaphysis, metaphysis, epiphysis, subarticular, cortex or medulla);
- density (sclerotic, lytic or mixed);
- borders – zone of transition well defined (narrow) or poorly defined;
- bony change – expansion, coarsened trabeculae, moth eaten (irregular holes also termed permeative lucency), osteopenia;
- periosteal reaction – lamellar, spiculated (tends to be associated with aggressive processes and can be hair on end, e.g. Ewing sarcoma, or sunray, e.g. metastases).

This patient's lesion is a solitary sclerotic cortical lesion with benign appearance and, in this age group, a healing fibrous cortical defect is most likely. The differential includes osteoid osteoma (particularly with a central lucency or nidus). Less likely is a bone infarct (check for history of sickle cell disease, steroids), bone island or fibrous dysplasia. Unlikely is metastasis (age, appearance), primary bone sarcoma or osteomyelitis (typically aggressive periosteal reaction).

A fibrous cortical defect (or non-ossifying fibroma if greater than 2 cm) is the most frequent benign bony lesion in children and adolescents. These lesions are developmental abnormalities and usually an incidental finding on radiographs. The lesion develops in the distal metaphysis of a long bone as a radiolucent and eccentrically located lesion, with thin cortex and sclerotic or scalloped margins while the growth plate is open. There is typically spontaneous healing with sclerosis once the growth plate has ossified. Surgery is considered if there is risk of a fracture (occupying greater than 50 per cent of the transverse diameter), symptoms or enlargement.

KEY POINTS

- A good description of the lesion helps with deriving a differential diagnosis.
- Age is one of the main discriminators in deciding differentials.

History

A 45-year-old man slipped and fell backwards onto his outstretched right arm. He presents complaining of severe shoulder pain and loss of movement. The shoulder is also swollen.

Examination

The patient holds his arm in slight abduction and external rotation. The shoulder is 'squared off' (i.e. box-like) with loss of deltoid contour compared with opposite side. The humeral head is just palpable anteriorly below the clavicle in the subcoracoid area. A careful assessment is made to check his radial pulses for a vascular injury and the axillary nerve function for regimental badge sensory loss over the deltoid and deltoid contraction on attempted abduction. Plain images are taken of the shoulder (Figure 38.1).

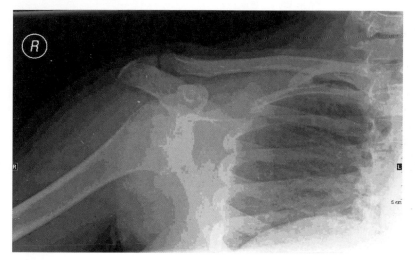

Figure 38.1 Posterior–anterior (PA) view of the right shoulder.

Questions

- What differential diagnoses should you consider?
- What complications can arise?
- What further imaging would be helpful?

The history and examination all suggest an anterior shoulder dislocation. Often in the case of trauma, shoulder injuries have to be assessed initially on the basis of a PA projection, which in this case confirms displacement of the humeral head inferiorly relative to the glenoid. Axial and Y views are nearly perpendicular to the PA projection and show the position of the humeral head. Figure 38.2 shows the humeral head anterior to the glenoid.

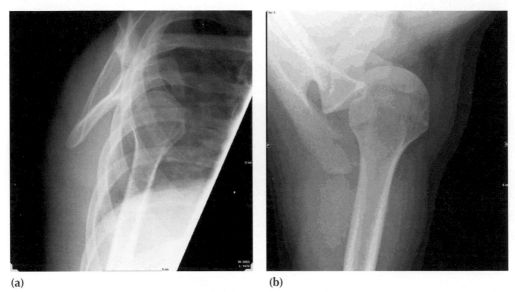

(a)   **(b)**

Figure 38.2 (a) Y view facing the glenoid fossa with the scapula describing a Y; (b) axial view of the right shoulder.

The imaging helps to distinguish the differential diagnosis of glenohumeral dislocation, of which anterior dislocation (96 per cent) is much more frequent than posterior (3 per cent) and inferior (1 per cent). Pseudo dislocation, where the humeral head is subluxed but not consistently dislocated, is associated with chronic shoulder joint instability, brachial plexus injury or haemarthrosis. Acromioclavicular dislocation and sternoclavicular dislocation should also be considered although much less common.

Posterior dislocations characteristically occur in trauma or seizure and can be harder to recognize, particularly if an axial or Y view has not been obtained. Suspicious features include fixed internal rotation (lightbulb sign), widening of the glenohumeral joint space (rim sign) with loss of overlap of the humerus over the glenoid.

Anterior dislocation can be associated with fracture of the greater tuberosity, anterior tear of the glenoid labrum (Bankart lesion), fracture of the anterior rim of the glenoid and an impaction fracture of the posterolateral surface of the humeral head (Hill–Sachs lesion) where it impacts on the glenoid rim. If not identified, recurrent dislocations are likely. The rotator cuff muscles may also be injured by traction.

Treatment requires adequate analgesia and sedation before relocating the joint. Imaging and neurovascular examination is performed before and after reduction.

Magnetic resonance (MR) is the investigation of choice to follow up a shoulder dislocation, particularly in younger patients who are more at risk of recurrent dislocations. Contrast injection into the joint (an arthrogram) may be required to see labral injuries reliably.

 KEY POINTS

- Anterior dislocations are much the commonest type of shoulder dislocation.
- Two views are required to identify dislocation, particularly posterior dislocations.
- The risk of recurrent dislocations increases with younger age and further imaging with MR may be required.

History

A 75-year-old man is brought to his general practice by his daughter. He complains of left-sided chest pain on inspiration. On further questioning it becomes apparent that he has had a recent fall. He lives alone and independently with frequent visits from his daughter who is concerned that there have been several falls. The patient is on blood pressure medication and takes a statin for previously high cholesterol. Reviewing his notes you see a previous attendance 2 years earlier for a fall and several episodes of treatment for pneumonia. There is a past history of smoking but no other significant medical history.

Examination

The observations are normal. He is thin. There is some bruising over the left side of the thorax and a notable low thoracic kyphosis. There are bilateral fine inspiratory crackles. The heart sounds are normal. The abdomen is unremarkable and no neurological or significant cognitive abnormality is noted.

A chest radiograph (Figure 39.1), electrocardiogram (ECG) and blood tests are arranged.

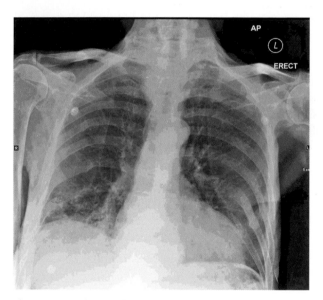

Figure 39.1 Chest radiograph.

Questions

- What does the radiograph show?
- What is the differential diagnosis?
- What further imaging would you consider?
- What other investigations should you consider?

ANSWER 39

Although the history and examination make rib fractures very likely, radiology is rarely indicated simply to look for low energy traumatic rib fractures. In this patient's case there are questions as to the cause of the fall. A chest radiograph is indicated for a possible chest infection or lesion and a thoracolumbar spine radiograph for the possible cause of the kyphosis.

The chest radiograph shows recent fractures of the left sixth to ninth ribs posterolaterally. There are also old fractures of the right ribs posterolaterally. Features that are common in trauma are fractures in a line and a posterolateral position, although this will depend on the type of trauma. Old fractures have healed and the bone cortex is continuous but the rib may be distorted. Recent and new fractures have discontinuous cortex but recent fractures show signs of healing with callus and bone remodelling that is absent in new fractures.

Do not stop looking once you have seen the fractures! Also look for other fractures (e.g. spine), bone lesions and examine the lungs, pleura and heart. On this radiograph there is consolidation in the right lower zone and a probable hiatus hernia gas bubble behind the heart.

The spine radiograph reported wedge compression fractures of the T11 and T12 vertebral bodies together with some small sclerotic and lytic lesions in the lumbar vertebrae. The initial blood tests show iron deficiency anaemia and raised erythrocyte sedimentation rate (ESR). This suggests an underlying systemic disease that affects bone and includes bowel or chest malignancy with bone metastases, myeloma or prostate carcinoma. The patient should be referred to the older person team for further investigation. From an imaging point of view this probably includes a computed tomography (CT) scan of the chest, abdomen and pelvis, although a bone scan could be helpful if sclerotic bone metastases from prostate or bowel carcinoma are suspected.

If blood tests suggest myeloma, a skeletal survey for lytic lesions could be done. Bone scans have lower sensitivity for lytic bone lesions which appear as photopenic regions of reduced uptake. The tracer used in bone scans, ^{99}Tc-MDP (technetium-99 conjugated with methylene diphosphonate), is taken up primarily by osteoblastic activity typical in sclerotic bone lesions.

The National Service Framework for older person care recommends a formal falls assessment in patients at risk and regular medication review.

 KEY POINTS

- Radiology is rarely indicated simply to look for rib fractures.
- In older patients the 'Occam's razor' approach of assuming only one underlying pathology has to be modified to allow for several interacting pathologies.
- Avoid 'satisfaction of search' and keep looking after spotting the first abnormality.

History

A 57-year-old man presents to his general practitioner (GP) with pain and swelling of his left big toe. He reported that this had been a longstanding problem over the last 7 years but had just put it down to 'old age' and did not want to trouble his GP with it. The pain and swelling would come and go in waves. He noted, however, that these episodes were now more frequent and he would struggle to weight bear on that side at times. On this occasion the pain had suddenly started at night and had been getting worse in flares ever since. In his past medical history he had a hernia operation 14 years ago. He was on treatment for hypertension and hyperlipidaemia with bendroflumethiazide and simvastatin, respectively. He is an ex-smoker and drinks 14 units of alcohol per week. He is not aware of any history of trauma.

Examination

Examination revealed a tender, erythematous right big toe with a markedly reduced range of motion at the first metatarsophalangeal joint. He had a moderately raised white cell count of 12 and his erythrocyte sedimentation rate (ESR) was also raised. Serum urate levels were elevated. He was afebrile and observations were otherwise normal. Radiographs of the foot were taken (Figure 40.1).

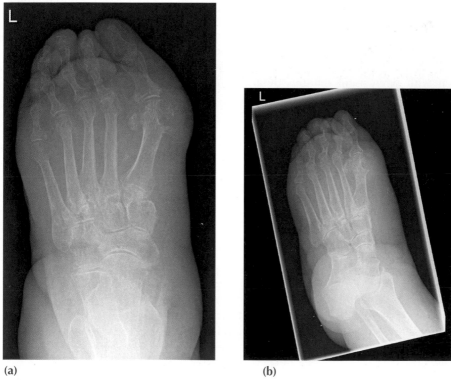

(a)   (b)

Figure 40.1 (a) Anterior–posterior and (b) oblique radiographs of the foot.

Questions

• What do the radiographs of the foot demonstrate?

Figure 40.1 demonstrates 'punched-out' lytic bone lesions with overhanging edges involving the first metatarsophalangeal joint with marginal sclerosis. There is the appearance of 'rat bites' with an overlying calcified soft-tissue swelling. These classical findings are consistent with longstanding gout.

Gout is defined as a peripheral arthritis that results from the deposition of sodium urate crystals in one or more joints. It has many contributing factors, but two central processes are involved in its development: the overproduction of uric acid and the underexcretion of uric acid. A multitude of conditions, including renal disease, have been implicated, but the vast majority of cases are idiopathic. Podagra (another name for pain in the first metatarsophalangeal joint) is the classic presentation of gout. In general, the symptoms of gout appear suddenly at night and occur in men with hyperuricaemia who are aged 30–60 years.

Gout is also associated with hyperlipidaemia, hypertension, kidney failure, obesity and insulin resistance. Other 'social' factors such as alcohol intake also increase the risk of gout. An increase in uric acid levels and resulting precipitation of gout is a side effect of thiazide diuretics.

Patients with new onset of acute gout usually have no radiographic findings and the classic features seen in this case are usually not seen until 6–12 years after initial attack. Early radiologic findings in gout are limited to the soft tissues and involve asymmetric swelling in the affected joints. There is preservation of joint space initially. In the intermediate stage of disease, gout causes subtle changes in the bony structures on plain film radiographs. In the periphery of affected joints, small 'punched-out' lytic bone lesions arise, often with sclerosis of margin. Obtaining two views is important to appreciate these subtle findings. Definitive diagnosis is made by finding the negatively birefringent crystals on polarized microscopy of synovial fluid aspirate.

The hallmark sign of late-phase gout is the appearance of large and numerous interosseous tophi on plain film radiographs. Calcific deposits in gouty tophi are seen in approximately 50 per cent of cases (only calcium urate crystals are opaque) and 'mouse/rat bite' erosions develop due to longstanding soft tissue tophi. Joint space narrowing and cartilage destruction is seen late in the course of the disease.

 KEY POINTS

- Classical plain radiographic features of longstanding gout include 'punched-out' lytic bone lesions with overhanging edges, marginal sclerosis and the appearance of 'rat bites' with an overlying calcified soft tissue swelling (tophus).
- These features usually are not usually seen until several years after initial attack and are present in around 50 per cent of patients.

CASE 41: A YOUNG MAN WITH PROGRESSIVE DYSPNOEA ON EXERTION

History

A 38-year-old man presents to his general practitioner (GP) with progressive dyspnoea on exertion developing steadily over the past 2 months. He says that he is now unable to walk 100 m before becoming severely short of breath and having to stop. He also noted the development of a non-productive cough over a similar time scale and more recently developing a fever. He had never experienced anything like this before and was previously fit and well with no past medical history of note. In his social history he reported having unprotected sex with both men and women.

Examination

On examination his respiratory rate was 22 per minute, fever (with a temperature of 37.9°C), a few crackles and wheezes over both lung fields. On the basis of the examination the GP sent the patient to the accident and emergency department.

In casualty, oxygen saturation was 90 per cent breathing air. Haematology results showed a normal white cell count. Biochemistry and liver function tests were normal. A retroviral screen showed he was human immunodeficiency virus (HIV) positive with a CD4 count below 200 cells/μL, consistent with acquired immune deficiency syndrome (AIDS). He was referred for a chest radiograph (Figure 41.1), on the basis of which a computed tomography (CT) was requested and performed (Figure 41.2).

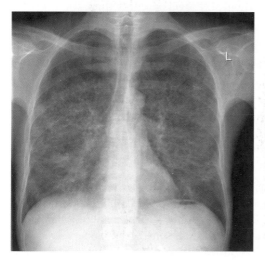

Figure 41.1 Chest radiograph.

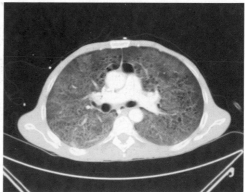

Figure 41.2 CT scan.

Questions

• What is the likely cause of his increasing shortness of breath?
• What do the chest radiograph (Figure 41.1) and subsequent CT scan (Figure 41.2) show?

121

The most likely diagnosis based on the clinical history and imaging findings is pneumocystis pneumonia (PCP) or pneumocystosis, which is a form of pneumonia, caused by the yeast-like fungus *Pneumocystis jirovecii*. The older name *Pneumocystis carinii* (which now only applies to the *Pneumocystis* variant that occurs in animals) is still in common usage.

Plain chest radiograph (Figure 41.1) demonstrates perihilar interstitial reticular shadowing with cyst formation. There is relative sparing of the apices and both bases. The axial enhanced CT image at the level of the pulmonary trunk (Figure 41.2) demonstrates perihilar ground-glass change and cystic changes, indicating the development of pneumatoceles.

Pneumocystis organisms are commonly found in the lungs of healthy individuals. It is believed most children have been exposed to the organism by the age of 4 years, and its occurrence is worldwide. The organism is a rare cause of infection in the general population, however it is a frequent cause of morbidity and mortality in persons who are immunocompromised, especially patients with AIDS.

Patients who do not have AIDS but are immunocompromised and at risk for PCP include individuals with haematologic malignancies, organ transplant recipients and those receiving long-term steroid or cytotoxic therapy, including patients with systemic vasculitis or other autoimmune deficiency. Other patients with immune deficiency disorders who are at particular risk for PCP include those with thymic dysplasia, those with severe combined immunodeficiency, and those with hypogammaglobulinaemia. Severe malnutrition may also predispose individuals to PCP.

The risk of pneumonia due to PCP increases when CD4 levels are less than 200 cells/μL.

The symptoms of PCP are non-specific. PCP in patients with HIV infection tends to run a more subacute, indolent course and tends to present much later, often after several weeks of symptoms, compared with PCP associated with other immunocompromising conditions.

Chest radiographs should be included in the initial evaluation for PCP. Frequently, these are the only images required. Characteristically, the distribution is central in location with bilateral diffuse symmetric finely granular, reticular interstitial/airspace infiltrates with perihilar and basilar distribution. Chest radiograph is normal in 10–39 per cent of patients with PCP. Hilar lymphadenopathy and pleural effusions are uncommon (seen in less than 5 per cent).

CT (in particular, high-resolution CT) scanning is more sensitive than chest radiography for the detection and exclusion of PCP pneumonia, and the results may be positive when chest radiograph findings are normal. CT findings include patchwork pattern bilateral asymmetric patchy mosaic appearance with sparing of segments/subsegments of pulmonary lobe or a 'ground-glass' pattern as in this case with bilateral diffuse airspace disease (fluid + inflammatory cells in alveolar space) in symmetric distribution. Cysts are visible on chest radiographs in 10 per cent of patients, although these are appreciated far more commonly on HRCT scans (33 per cent). Findings of cysts or pneumatoceles are not infrequent in patients with PCP.

KEY POINTS

- PCP is the most common cause of interstitial pneumonia in immunocompromised patients, which quickly leads to airspace disease.
- Chest radiograph findings may be normal in a significant number of patients with PCP.
- The classical chest radiograph features of PCP pneumonia, when present, are bilateral, diffuse, often perihilar, fine, reticular interstitial opacification, which appears to be granular.

History

A 67-year-old man presents to the accident and emergency department as a referral from his general practitioner (GP). Over the course of the preceding 12 hours he has been experiencing pain in the left side of his chest, worst on deep inspiration. This is the first ever such episode and he describes the pain as sharp and stabbing. He is an ex-smoker with a 30 pack-year history. Emphysematous changes have been noted on a previous chest radiograph and he takes a salbutamol inhaler as required along with an inhaled corticosteroid regularly. Aside from a history of mild to moderate chronic obstructive pulmonary disease he was otherwise well. He denies any history of trauma.

Examination

He is tachypnoeic with a respiratory rate of 33/minute and tachycardic with a heart rate of 104/minute which electrocardiogram (ECG) confirms as sinus rhythm with no acute changes. On examination of the respiratory system there is reduced expansion, a slightly hyperresonant percussion note and reduced air entry on the left. Vocal resonance is also reduced on the left. No added sounds are identified, however. Full blood count (FBC), biochemistry and liver function tests are all normal. Blood gas analysis demonstrates a Pa_{O_2} of 9 kPa with a Pa_{CO_2} of 4.5 kPa. The patient is referred for a chest radiograph (Figure 42.1).

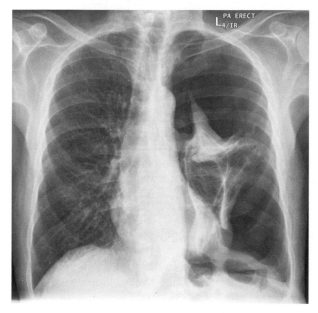

Figure 42.1 Posterior–anterior (PA) chest radiograph.

Questions

- What abnormality do you see on the chest radiograph?
- What concerning features would you look for?
- How would you manage this patient?

ANSWER 42

The PA chest radiograph (Figure 42.1) shows a large left pneumothorax, which appears tethered to the left costal pleura. There is a background of emphysematous change but no evidence of mediastinal shift to suggest that the pneumothorax is under tension, which would be an alarming feature requiring immediate intervention.

Pneumothorax refers to the presence of air within the pleural space. Diagnosis is established on the plain chest radiograph by demonstrating an outer margin of the visceral pleura known as the pleural line (delineating collapsed lung), separated from the parietal pleura (chest wall) by a lucent space occupied by gas and devoid of any pulmonary markings.

The pleural line demonstrating the margin of collapsed lung can sometimes be difficult to detect in cases of a small pneumothorax. It is important to note that a skin fold may mimic the pleural line. When a pneumothorax is suspected but not confirmed on inspiratory radiograph, an expiratory image may confirm the diagnosis. This is because at the end of expiration, the constant volume of the gas within the pneumothorax is accentuated by the reduction of the hemithorax.

Chest radiography is the first investigation performed to assess pneumothorax, because it is straightforward, rapid, cheap and non-invasive. CT may be used in more complex cases, for example in planning pleurodesis (usually in recurrent pneumothoraces) and it is more sensitive than plain radiographs in detecting blebs or bullae or a small pneumothorax.

Pneumothorax is classified as spontaneous (atraumatic), traumatic, or iatrogenic:

- **Spontaneous pneumothorax** may be either primary (occurring in persons without clinically or radiologically apparent lung disease) or secondary (in which lung disease is present and apparent, as in this example). Most individuals with primary spontaneous pneumothorax have unrecognized lung disease; it is often thought to occur due to rupture of a subpleural bleb.
- **Traumatic pneumothorax** is caused by penetrating or blunt trauma to the chest. Gas enters the pleural space directly through the chest wall through visceral pleural penetration or alveolar rupture resulting from sudden compression of the chest.
- **Iatrogenic pneumothorax** results from a complication of a diagnostic or therapeutic intervention. With the increasing use of invasive diagnostic procedures, iatrogenic pneumothorax has become more common.

In this large secondary pneumothorax with significant symptoms drainage is required to remove the air from the pleural space. Needle aspiration is not usually adequate in such cases and insertion of an intercostal drain is required. This has been done in Figure 42.2 with some resulting but as yet incomplete re-expansion of the collapsed left lung.

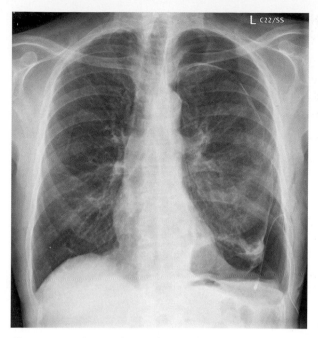

Figure 42.2 Chest radiograph post drainage.

 KEY POINTS

- In the erect position, pleural gas collects over the apex where the space between the lung and the chest wall is most notable.
- It is important to assess for radiographic manifestations of tension pneumothorax are mediastinal shift, diaphragmatic depression and rib cage expansion.
- Tension pneumothorax is an emergency requiring immediate intervention.

History

A 45-year-old woman attends the accident and emergency department following a fall off a stepladder from a height of 1 metre onto her outstretched right arm while decorating at home. She immediately noted marked pain and is unable to flex or extend the elbow joint. She is previously fit and well, with no previous illnesses. She is right hand dominant.

Examination

She is unable to pronate or supinate the forearm and unable to flex or extend the elbow. She demonstrates bony tenderness maximal over the radial head and there is swelling of the elbow joint. Her arm pulses are intact distally, capillary refill is less than 2 seconds, and sensation and power in the hand and wrist are normal. Plain radiographs are taken (Figure 43.1a,b).

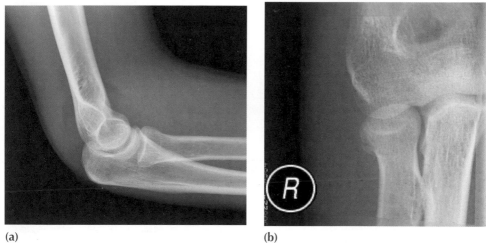

(a)   (b)

Figure 43.1 (a) Lateral and (b) magnified anterior–posterior (AP) images.

Question

- What is the likely injury?
- What do the plain radiographs show?

ANSWER 43

The lateral radiograph (Figure 43.1a) demonstrates elevated anterior and posterior elbow fat pads, suggesting a joint effusion and is suspicious for an occult fracture. The magnified AP image (Figure 43.1b) confirms a fracture of the radial head.

The preferred study for the evaluation of elbow trauma is conventional radiography and the radiographic examination requires the acquisition of two views: the lateral view, ideally in 90 degree flexion, and AP view in full extension.

The classic elbow 'fat pad' sign seen on lateral elbow radiograph is an invaluable soft tissue finding in cases of intra-articular injury of the elbow. Fat is normally present within the joint capsule of the elbow, but outside the synovium. As it is usually 'hidden' in the concavity of the olecranon and coronoid fossae, fat is usually not visible on the lateral radiograph.

Injuries causing intra-articular haemorrhage/effusion, however, cause distension of the synovium which forces the fat out of the fossa, producing triangular radiolucent shadows anterior and posterior to the distal end of the humerus – the radiographic sail sign (Figure 43.2).

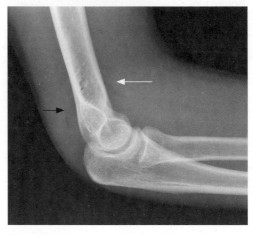

The posterior fat pad (black arrow – Figure 43.2) is not normally seen on radiographs and its presence is always an abnormal finding that requires further investigation for an occult fracture.

The anterior fat pad may be normally visualized on lateral radiographs as a triangular radiolucency, although in the presence of joint effusion it is displaced anteriorly, becoming more pronounced and the anterior margin becomes convex. Fat pad signs may not be evident if the fracture is extracapsular.

Fracture of the radial head is the most common type of elbow fracture in adults, whereas fractures of the radial neck are more common in children. Fractures of the

Figure 43.2

radial head and neck of the radius generally result from a hard fall on an outstretched hand with the impact of fall driving the head of radius axially onto the capitulum of the humerus.

Treatment depends on the degree of displacement, angulation and articular involvement. Minor degrees such as that shown are often treated by early mobilization in a brace to minimize later elbow stiffness.

 KEY POINTS

- Radiographic examination requires two views: AP view in full extension and lateral view, ideally in 90 degrees of flexion.
- The posterior fat pad is not normally seen on radiographs, and its presence is always an abnormal finding that should prompt further investigation for occult fractures.
- Fat pad signs may not be evident if the fracture is extracapsular.

History

A 22-year-old man attends the accident and emergency department following a fight. He remembers punching another man and, although intoxicated, is complaining of pain in the knuckles. He is otherwise fit and well.

Examination

On examination his knuckles are swollen and tender to palpation. There is maximal tenderness in the region of the fifth metacarpal head (base of the little finger) with virtually no range of movement at the fifth metacarpophalangeal joint. Neurovascular function is intact distally. Plain radiographs are taken (Figure 44.1).

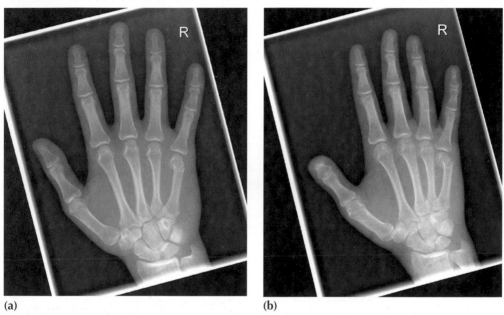

(a)   (b)

Figure 44.1 (a) Anterior–posterior (AP) and (b) oblique plain radiographs.

Questions
- What is the likely injury?
- Describe the injury seen in the plain radiographs of the hand.

ANSWER 44

The AP and oblique images of the hand demonstrate a metacarpal neck fracture, with volar angulation and displacement of the distal fragment. Note also prominent soft tissue swelling of the hand.

A 'boxer's fracture' is the common name for a fracture involving the neck of the fifth metacarpal, which forms the knuckle of the little finger (but the same name may also be used for a fracture at the neck of any of the metacarpals). It is usually caused by the impact of a clenched fist with a skull or a hard, immovable object.

Only the collateral ligaments remain attached to the proximal phalanx and therefore the metacarpal head is freed from any proximal stabilizing influence. The metacarpal head tilts volarly, causing the joint to lie in hyperextension and the collateral ligaments become slack. If the joint is allowed to remain in hyperextension, collateral ligaments will shorten, leading to limited metacarpophalangeal flexion.

The little finger carpometacarpal articulation allows a flexion–extension arc of 20–30 degrees in addition to a rotatory motion, facilitating little finger opposition to thumb.

A true lateral radiograph is necessary with these fractures in order to measure the angle of displacement of the distal fragment. The normal metacarpal neck angle is about 15 degrees and therefore a measured angle on film of 30 degrees is actually approximately 15 degrees.

These fractures are often angulated, and if severely so, require pins to be put in place and realignment as well as the usual splinting. However, the prognosis on these fractures is generally good.

 KEY POINTS

- A boxer's fracture is the common name for a break in the end of the little finger metacarpal bone, also known as a fifth metacarpal fracture.
- The injury is commonly caused by punching something harder than the hand, for example, a wall. The end of the metacarpal bone takes the brunt of the impact, which usually breaks through the neck (which is the narrowest area near the end) and bends down toward the palm.

History

A 20-year-old man attends the accident and emergency department following a fall onto his flexed left wrist while playing football.

Examination

He demonstrates a markedly reduced range of movement and is complaining of point tenderness on the dorsum and ulnar aspect of the left wrist. There is no pain on palpation of the anatomical snuffbox or upon axial loading of the thumb. Radiographs are taken (Figures 45.1 and 45.2).

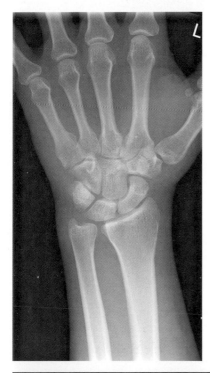

Figure 45.1 (a) Anterior–posterior (AP) view of the left wrist.

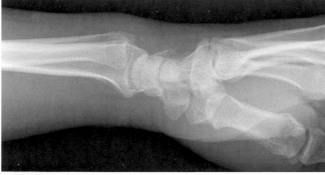

Figure 45.2 Lateral view of the left wrist.

Questions
- What injury do you suspect he may have sustained?
- What do the wrist radiographs demonstrate?

Triquetral fractures typically occur from a hyperextension injury with the wrist in ulnar deviation, however, can also occur with hyperflexion. Either the dorsal or volar radiotriquetral ligaments may avulse triquetral fragments at their attachments. Behind fractures of the scaphoid, triquetral fractures are the second most common carpal bone to fracture. They are frequently seen as dorsal chip fractures only on the lateral projection (Figure 45.2) since the pisiform usually overlies the triquetrum on the frontal projection of the wrist (Figure 45.1). In this case there is a small avulsion from the dorsum of the triquetrum seen only on the lateral projection (arrow, Figure 45.3).

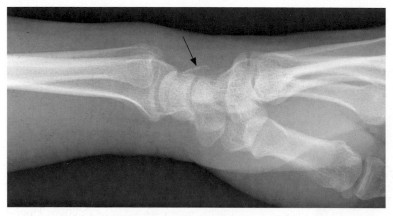

Figure 45.3 Lateral view of the left wrist indicating the fracture.

Patients will usually complain of localized tenderness on the dorsum of the wrist.

The triquetrum may be identified by its pyramidal shape and by an oval isolated facet for articulation with the pisiform bone. It is situated just distal to the ulna and the triangular fibrocartilage complex, proximal to the base of the hamate.

The superior surface presents a medial, rough, non-articular portion, and a lateral convex articular portion, which articulates with the triangular articular disc of the wrist. The inferior surface, directed laterally, is concave, sinuously curved and smooth for articulation with the hamate. The dorsal surface is rough for the attachment of ligaments. The triquetrum articulates on its radial side with the lunate to which it is attached by the lunotriquetral ligament. On the volar (palmar) aspect there is an articulation with the pisiform.

Triquetral fractures may divided into two types:

- **Chip fractures:** A chip fracture, usually off the dorsal radial surface, typically occurs with a wrist hyperextension injury. Chip fractures can also occur with the hyperflexion.
- **Mid-body fracture:** Fractures through the mid-body of the triquetrum are less frequent than a chip fracture. This type of fracture is usually due to a direct blow, or may occur in conjunction with a perilunate dislocation. The dislocation may have been reduced, so a triquetral fracture from the proximal radial aspect of the bone may indicate the presence of a former dislocation.

 KEY POINTS

- Triquetral fractures are the second most common fracture of the carpal bones.
- They are frequently seen as dorsal chip fractures only on the lateral projection as the pisiform usually overlies the triquetrum on the AP projection of the wrist.

History

A 55-year-old man is admitted to the accident and emergency department complaining of gradual onset of shortness of breath over the course of several hours along with right-sided chest pain aggravated by deep inspiration. He is complaining of mild lightheadedness and feels the symptoms are getting worse. The pain is sharp and stabbing in nature. He was previously fit and well. One day earlier he returned on a long haul flight from a business trip to Asia. He denies any history of leg swelling.

Examination

Upon admission to hospital his oxygen saturation on air was 94 per cent and his respiratory rate was 20/minute. A chest radiograph failed to demonstrate any focal lesion. Routine bloods were normal although D-dimer performed in the emergency department was elevated. Electrocardiogram (ECG) demonstrated a mild sinus tachycardia heart rate of only 102/minute. The accident and emergency team suspected a possible pulmonary embolism (PE) and so a computed tomography pulmonary angiogram (CTPA) was performed (Figures 46.1 and 46.2).

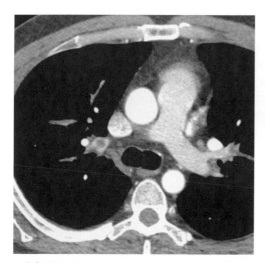
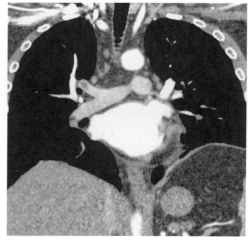

Axial CTPA image.

Figure 46.2 Reformatted coronal CTPA image.

Question

- What do the CT images demonstrate?

ANSWER 46

Figures 46.1 and 46.2 demonstrate axial and reformatted coronal CTPA images respectively, showing a large filling defect within the distal right main pulmonary artery extending into the upper lobe artery.

The initial chest radiograph in patients with pulmonary embolism is frequently normal. An initially normal chest radiograph may over time begin to show atelectasis, which can progress to cause a small pleural effusion and an elevated hemidiaphragm. After 24–72 hours, one third of patients with proven PE develop focal infiltrates that are indistinguishable from an infectious pneumonia. Occasionally, there may be evidence of Westermark sign, which is focal oligaemia (absence of blood vessel markings) beyond the location of the pulmonary embolism and dilatation of those vessels proximally. A rare late finding of pulmonary infarction is the Hampton hump, a triangular or rounded pleural-based infiltrate with the apex pointed toward the hilum, frequently located adjacent to the diaphragm.

CTPA is the most common study used for detection of pulmonary embolism and has become accepted both as the preferred primary diagnostic modality and as the standard for making or excluding the diagnosis of PE. In the majority of patients, multi-detector CT scans with intravenous contrast can resolve third-order pulmonary vessels.

It is important to note, however, that multi-detector CTPA carries a radiation dose and can miss lesions in a patient with pleuritic chest pain due to multiple small emboli that have lodged in distal vessels. In patients with a normal chest radiograph, nuclear scintigraphic ventilation–perfusion (V/Q) scanning of the lung is an alternative diagnostic modality for detecting PE with a lower radiation dose. This modality is recommended only for patients with a normal chest radiograph in order to prevent spurious perfusion mismatch from other lung processes.

 KEY POINTS

- The initial chest radiograph in patients with PE is frequently normal.
- CTPA is the most common study used for detection of PE and has become accepted both as the preferred primary diagnostic modality and as the standard for making or excluding the diagnosis of PE.
- It is important to note, however, that in patients with a normal chest radiograph, ventilation–perfusion (V/Q) scanning is an alternative modality carrying a lower radiation dose.

History

A 40-year-old man arrives in the United Kingdom from Bangladesh to visit relatives. He has been complaining of feeling generally unwell with a cough and fever for around 3 weeks, which is worsening. He attends the accident and emergency department complaining of a productive cough and feels increasingly systemically unwell with fevers and sweating. He has has been well previously with no smoking history or history of exposure to dust.

Examination

His respiratory rate is 24 per minute and pulse 92 per minute. On respiratory examination there is limited expansion with resonance to percussion, rather quiet breath sounds but no bronchial breathing and no added sounds. He is febrile with a temperature of 40°C. Oxygen saturation is 92 per cent breathing air. Full blood count shows a white cell count of $20 \times 10^3/mm^3$.

He is admitted to hospital under the care of the medical team but after a further 24 hours, the intensive care team are asked to review the patient as his breathing and oxygenation have deteriorated further. He is intubated and transferred to the intensive care unit where central lines and a nasogastric tube are inserted. A chest radiograph is performed (Figure 47.1) and, based on this, a computed tomography (CT) scan of the chest was requested (Figure 47.2).

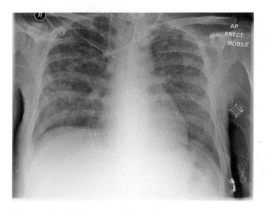

Figure 47.1 Chest radiograph.

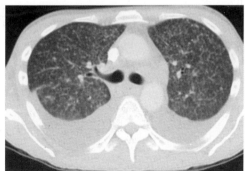

Figure 47.2 Axial CT image.

Questions

- Ignoring the bilateral internal jugular lines, what are the lung changes on the chest radiograph in Figure 47.1?
- How would you describe the pattern of disease on CT (Figure 47.2)?

The initial chest radiograph (Figure 47.1) shows diffuse patchy consolidation on a background of widespread tiny nodules distributed throughout all lobes bilaterally. Subsequent CT (Figure 47.2) confirms the presence of randomly distributed, diffuse tiny nodules and bilateral large pleural effusions. Findings are suggestive of miliary tuberculosis.

Miliary tuberculosis (TB) is the widespread dissemination of *Mycobacterium tuberculosis* via hematogenous spread. Classic miliary TB is defined as 'millet like' (approximately 2 mm) seeding of TB bacilli in the lung, as evidenced on chest radiography. This pattern is seen in 1–3 per cent of all TB cases.

Following exposure and inhalation of TB bacilli in the lung, a primary pulmonary complex is established, followed by development of pulmonary lymphangitis and hilar lymphadenopathy. Mycobacteraemia and haematogenous seeding occur after the primary infection. After initial inhalation of TB bacilli, miliary TB may occur as primary TB or may develop years after the initial infection. The disseminated nodules consist of central caseating necrosis and peripheral epithelioid and fibrous tissue.

Imaging findings may take weeks between the time of dissemination and the radiographic appearance of disease. Up to 30 per cent have a normal chest radiograph. When first visible, the nodules measure about 1 mm in size, but they can grow to 2–3 mm if left untreated. High-resolution CT scans are more sensitive at demonstrating small nodules. Nodules are either sharply or poorly defined and around 1–4 mm in size in a diffuse, random distribution. There may be associated intra- and interlobular septal thickening.

Radiographically, nodules are not calcified, as opposed to the initial Ghon focus, which is often visible on chest radiographs as a small calcified nodule. Chest CT scanning is useful in the presence of suggestive and inconclusive chest radiography findings. When treated, clearing is frequently rapid. Under the age of 5 years, there is an increased risk of meningitis.

Risk factors include immunosuppression, cancer, transplantation, human immunodeficiency virus (HIV) infection, malnutrition, diabetes, silicosis and endstage renal disease.

 KEY POINTS

- Miliary TB is caused by the widespread haematogenous dissemination of *Mycobacterium tuberculosis*. It is so named because the nodules are the size of millet seeds (1–5 mm with a mean of 2 mm).
- Miliary TB represents only approximately 1–3 per cent of all cases of TB.
- It is considered to be a manifestation of primary TB, although clinical appearance of miliary TB may not occur for many years after initial infection.

History

A 33-year-old man was a passenger of car involved in a head-on collision travelling at 60 mph (97 km/h). He is brought into the accident and emergency department as a trauma call. He was sitting in the rear of the car in the central passenger seat restrained by an old-style 'lap belt', unlike the other passengers who were wearing standard shoulder and lap belts. He was thrown forward into the seat in front. He was conscious throughout but is complaining of severe pain in the lower thoracic and lumbar spine.

Examination

Primary survey is unremarkable and his observations are stable. There is marked tenderness over the lower thoracic and lumbar spine. On neurological examination of the lower limbs there are no motor or sensory abnormalities. Per rectal examination revealed normal tone. A computed tomography (CT) examination of the thorax and abdomen was obtained with sagittal (Figure 48.1a,b) and coronal (Figure 48.1c) reformats.

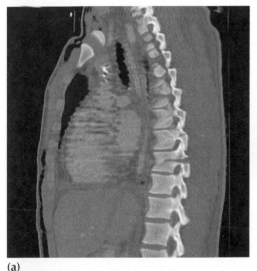
(a)

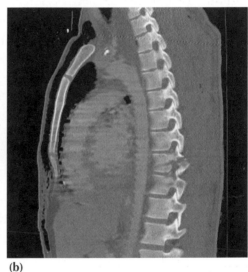
(b)

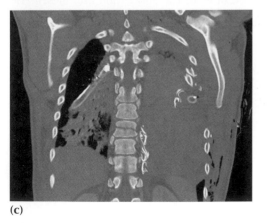
(c)

Question

• What abnormality do the CT images show?

Figure 48.1 CT scans: (a,b) sagittal and (c) coronal views.

ANSWER 48

The sagittal (Figure 48.1a,b) and coronal (Figure 48.1c) reformats of the spine show a 'Chance' fracture line extending through the spinous process, lamina, pedicles and vertebral body of T9 (a horizontal splitting of the vertebra beginning with the spinous process or lamina and extending anteriorly through the pedicles and vertebral body).

Chance fracture is caused by a flexion injury of the spine, first described by G.Q. Chance in 1948. It consists of a compression injury to the anterior portion of the vertebral body and a transverse fracture through the posterior elements of the vertebra and the posterior portion of the vertebral body. It is caused by violent forward flexion, causing distraction injury to the posterior elements.

Chance fractures later became known as 'seatbelt' fractures with the advent of lap seatbelts in cars. A head-on collision would cause the passenger wearing a lap belt to suddenly be flexed at the waist, hence creating significant stress on the posterior elements of the vertebra. From the 1980s when shoulder and lap belts became more common in cars Chance fractures have become less associated with road traffic accidents and are more commonly seen with falls or crush-type injuries where the thorax is acutely hyperflexed.

The most common site at which Chance fractures occur is the thoracolumbar junction and mid-lumbar region in paediatric populations.

An anterior–posterior (AP) view of the spine may reveal disruption of the pedicles and loss of vertebral body height. Frequently a transverse process fracture will be identified on AP projection. The lateral view will demonstrate the spinous process fracture and fractures through the laminae and pedicles. The vertebral body will usually look compressed and wedge shaped.

CT of the spine should be performed on all Chance fractures to assess the extent of the fracture and to evaluate the spinal canal. Sagittal reconstructions of the axial images provide a great deal of information about the fracture pattern. Posterior element fractures are better seen on lateral projection, although the AP view helps to demonstrate pedicle involvement.

Up to 50 per cent of Chance fractures have associated intra-abdominal injuries, including fractures of the pancreas, contusions or lacerations of the duodenum and mesenteric contusions or lacerations.

 KEY POINTS

- The incidence of associated intra-abdominal injuries with a Chance fracture reaches 50 per cent. Therefore, when a Chance fracture is diagnosed a CT of the abdomen should be obtained.
- Injuries associated with Chance fractures include fractures of the pancreas, duodenum and mesentery contusions/rupture.

History

A 30-year-old woman is admitted via the accident and emergency department with diffuse cramping abdominal pain. She has not opened her bowels for 4 days. She has a history of painful endometriosis and has been using increasing amounts of opiate analgesia to control the pain.

Examination

Her observations are all within the normal range. Her haematology and biochemistry results are also normal.

The abdomen is soft with no guarding or rebound tenderness. Bowels sounds are present and normal. Per rectal exam demonstrates a rectum containing solid stool.

A plain radiograph of the abdomen was performed (Figure 49.1).

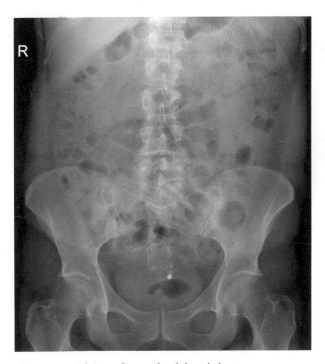

Figure 49.1 Plain radiograph of the abdomen.

Question

• What abnormalities can be seen in the abdomen radiograph?

ANSWER 49

The radiograph of the abdomen demonstrates faecal loading of the large bowel but no significantly dilated loops (Figure 49.1) There is no evidence of free gas or pneumoperitoneum. Projected over the mid pelvis is an intrauterine contraceptive device (IUCD) (arrow, Figure 49.2). These are frequently seen as an incidental findings in radiographs of the abdomen and pelvis. A piercing is also present.

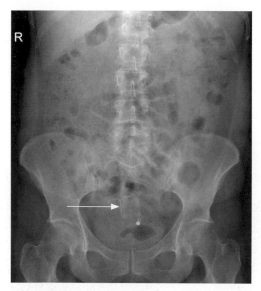

Figure 49.2

The IUCD is a form of birth control. It is an object, placed in the uterus, to prevent pregnancy. The aim of these devices is to confer long-term, reversible protection against unwanted pregnancy. They may, however, induce menstrual complications as well as an increased risk of pelvic inflammatory disease and ectopic pregnancy. They can also be spontaneously expelled from the uterus without being noticed by the patient.

Among modern IUCDs, the two types available are copper-containing devices and a hormone-containing device that releases a progestogen. Currently, there are several different kinds of copper IUCDs available in different parts of the world, and there is one hormonal device, called Mirena®.

An IUCD can increase the risk of spontaneous abortion unless removed in cases where intrauterine pregnancy occurs. Complications at the time of insertion include pain, syncope and uterine perforation.

In this case, however, the most likely cause of the patient's abdominal pain is constipation due to opiate analgesia use and the IUCD is an incidental finding.

 KEY POINTS

- Intrauterine contraceptive devices (IUCDs) are a commonly used form of birth control and are frequently seen as an incidental finding on radiographs.

History

A 66-year-old woman is admitted to the accident and emergency department with sudden onset of chest pain 1 hour earlier. She had otherwise been fit and well apart from a history of hypertension for which she had been treated with amlodipine for the last 11 years.

Examination

The electrocardiogram (ECG) shows evidence of left ventricular hypertrophy. Troponin was not raised. D-dimer was moderately elevated. A chest radiograph was performed (Figure 50.1). The accident and emergency team were concerned about the possibility of a pulmonary embolism and therefore a computed tomography pulmonary angiogram (CTPA) was performed (one axial slice is shown in Figure 50.2). No pulmonary embolism or focal lung parenchymal abnormality was seen.

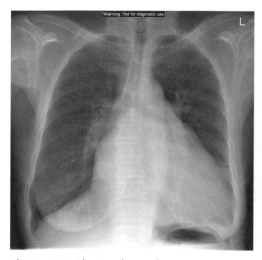

Figure 50.1 Chest radiograph.

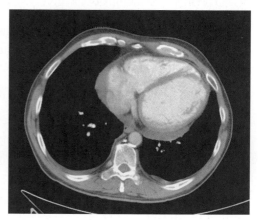

Figure 50.2 Axial CTPA image.

Question

- What abnormalities do the chest radiograph in Figure 50.1 and axial enhanced CT image (at the level of the heart) seen in Figure 50.2 demonstrate?

ANSWER 50

The chest radiograph (Figure 50.1) demonstrates that the heart is enlarged (there is cardiomegaly), shown by the fact that the cardiothoracic ratio is greater than 50 per cent on the posterior–anterior (PA) view. The cardiothoracic ratio is the maximum transverse diameter of the heart divided by the greatest internal diameter of the thoracic cage (from inside of rib to inside of rib). This is again demonstrated on the CTPA (in Figure 50.2). Cardiomegaly is often first detected on chest radiograph.

In normal people the cardiothoracic ratio is usually less than 50 per cent, measured by taking the maximum transverse diameter of the heart on a PA film as a proportion of the thoracic diameter at the same level. Therefore, the cardiothoracic ratio is a convenient way of separating most normal hearts from most abnormal hearts. The heart size should be assessed on every chest radiograph. On an AP film the cardiac size is magnified so a ratio over 50 per cent may not indicate cardiac enlargement. If the heart is enlarged, check for other signs of heart failure such as pulmonary oedema, septal (Kerley B) lines and pleural effusions.

A multitude of conditions can give rise to cardiomegaly, which is thought to result from the direct effect of the thickening of the heart muscles when the heart is given an increased workload. Causative factors include heart valve disorders, high blood pressure, severe anaemia, thyroid disorders, viral illnesses, drug abuse and previous heart attacks, which can cause the heart to overwork. An increase in workload, however, may also be caused by exercise.

 KEY POINTS

- If there is cardiomegaly, look for other signs of heart failure.
- Cardiomegaly may be the first sign of an occult systemic or cardiovascular disease.

CASE 51: A MIRROR IMAGE

History

A 41-year-old woman was transferred to high dependency unit (HDU) from the general medical ward where her breathing had been steadily deteriorating. She had been admitted with a short history of worsening dyspnoea and cough over 2 days. She had demonstrated pyrexia and raised inflammatory markers and had been treated with high flow oxygen and antibiotics for a presumed pneumonia but had continued to worsen. The patient was too unwell to give a medical history but no significant previous medical history had been noted by the admitting team.

Examination

On examination she is tachypnoic (30/minute) and there is bronchial breathing in both mid zones with inspiratory crackles in the same areas. Air entry was reduced bilaterally.

On examination for the heart sounds it is noted that they cannot be appreciated in the normal left praecordial position and the apex beat is also not palpable on the left. Instead the apex beat is palpated and heart sounds are auscultated on the right of the praecordium. Palpation of the abdomen suggests a liver edge under the left costophrenic angle.

Question

- What condition do you think the patient may have?
- What variations are there?
- What do the chest radiograph (Figure 51.1) and the axial enhanced computed tomography (CT) image (Figure 51.2) show.

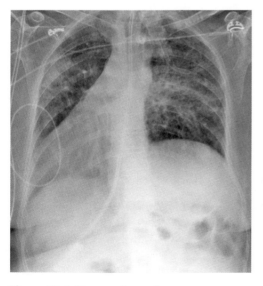

Figure 51.1 Chest radiograph.

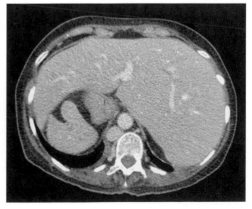

Figure 51.2 Axial enhanced CT image.

ANSWER 51

The chest radiograph in Figure 51.1 demonstrates that the heart is positioned within the right side of the chest (dextrocardia). There is bilateral patchy consolidation within both lungs, explaining the patient's respiratory deterioration, and a nasogastric tube inserted by the HDU team can be seen extending below the right hemithorax instead of the usual left. The CT scan (Figure 51.2) confirms that the liver and spleen are in opposite positions to normal, suggestive of situs inversus.

Situs inversus is present in approximately 0.01 per cent of the population. Also called situs transversus or oppositus, it is a congenital condition in which the major visceral organs are reversed or mirrored from their normal positions. The term 'situs inversus' is a short form of the Latin phrase *situs inversus viscerum*, meaning 'inverted position of the internal organs'. The normal arrangement is known as situs solitus. In other rare cases, in a condition known as situs ambiguous or heterotaxy, situs cannot be determined.

In situs inversus, the morphologic right atrium is on the left and the morphologic left atrium is on the right. The usual pulmonary anatomy is also reversed such that the left lung has three lobes and the right lung has two. Furthermore, the liver and gallbladder are located on the left, whereas the stomach and spleen are positioned on the right (as in the CT shown in Figure 51.2). The remaining internal structures are also a mirror image of the normal.

Isolated dextrocardia is also termed 'situs solitus with dextrocardia'. The cardiac apex points to the right but organs are otherwise in their usual positions. Situs inversus with dextrocardia is also termed 'situs inversus totalis' because the heart position, in addition to the atrial chambers and abdominal viscera, is a mirror image of the normal anatomy.

The classification of situs is independent of the cardiac apical position.

Approximately 20 per cent of patients with situs inversus have an underlying condition known as primary ciliary dyskinesia. This is a dysfunction of the cilia, which manifests during embryonic development. As normal cilia play a role in determining the position of internal organs during development, these individuals have a higher chance of developing situs inversus and Kartagener's syndrome, which is characterized by the triad of situs inversus, chronic sinusitis and bronchiectasis.

 KEY POINTS

- Situs inversus is a congenital condition in which the major visceral organs are reversed or mirrored from their normal positions.
- When situs cannot be determined, the patient has situs ambiguous or heterotaxy. In these patients, the liver may be midline, the spleen multiple or absent, the atrial morphology aberrant and the bowel malrotated. Frequently, normally unilateral structures are duplicated or absent.

CASE 52: A DISTENDED AND PAINFUL ABDOMEN

History

A 72-year-old woman presented to the accident and emergency department with increasing nausea, distension and crampy lower abdominal pain over the previous 2 weeks. Over a similar time course there has been bright red blood mixed in with her stools and a slight feeling of incomplete emptying after going to the toilet. There was no history of vomiting. She was normally very independent and had not wanted to bother her general practitioner (GP). However, the pain had become increasingly unbearable such that her husband called an ambulance.

Examination

She looked pale and dehydrated although her observations were all normal apart from mild postural hypotension. Her abdomen was distended, with generalized tenderness and voluntary guarding. The bowel sounds were tinkling and upon per rectal examination there was the impression of a hard mass. Full blood count revealed a mild microcytic anaemia, with haemoglobin 9.8 g/dL. A plain radiograph of the abdomen was performed in accident and emergency (Figure 52.1) and on the basis of this the surgical team requested computed tomography (CT) imaging (Figures 52.2 and 52.3).

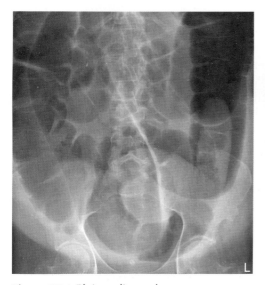

Figure 52.1 Plain radiograph.

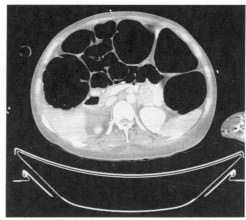

Figure 52.2 Axial CT scan.

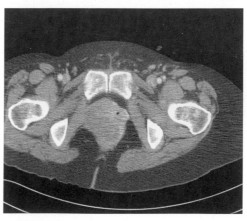

Figure 52.3 Axial CT scan.

Question

- What does the plain radiograph demonstrate?
- What is the differential diagnosis?
- What do the axial CT images show?

ANSWER 52

Figure 52.1 demonstrates multiple loops of dilated large bowel filling the abdomen consistent with a distal mechanical large bowel obstruction or pseudo-obstruction (note the radiograph is suboptimal as the upper abdomen has been missed). Figure 52.2 shows an axial contrast enhanced CT image on lung windows at the level of the adrenal glands demonstrating multiple dilated loops of large bowel distending the abdomen. Figure 52.3 with soft tissue CT windows demonstrates a large obstructing, circumferential bulky rectal mass as the cause of the large bowel obstruction.

The most common causes of mechanical large bowel obstruction in this age of patient would include colon cancer, diverticulitis or sigmoid volvulus. Less common causes of large bowel obstruction include inflammatory bowel disease, hernias, adhesions or endometriosis.

Approximately 25 per cent of all intestinal obstructions occur in the large bowel. Large bowel obstruction is a common emergency condition that requires early identification and intervention and may result from either mechanical interruption of the flow of intestinal contents or by the dilation of the colon in the absence of an anatomic lesion (pseudo-obstruction). Distinguishing between a true mechanical obstruction and a pseudo-obstruction is important as the treatment differs.

Radiologically, the large bowel is characterized on plain film by its haustrations and sacculations, which are most prominent in the ascending and transverse colon but can also be seen in the left colon. With moderate distention of the large bowel, the haustral folds appear to extend entirely across the lumen but this appearance may disappear with further distension. The haustral folds of the large bowel are more widely spaced than the valvulae conniventes of the small bowel. The large bowel will normally contain solid material, whereas small bowel usually contains liquid and gas only. Furthermore, large bowel tends to be peripherally located, whereas the small bowel is centrally located.

The colon is dilated when it exceeds 6 cm in diameter, and the caecum is dilated when it exceeds 9 cm. When the caecal diameter exceeds 10 cm the risk of perforation is high. The caecum always dilates to the largest extent no matter the location of large bowel obstruction.

Gas and faeces tend to accumulate proximal to the point of obstruction. In a typical configuration of mechanical obstruction, all colonic segments proximal to the point of luminal narrowing are dilated. In most cases of large bowel obstruction, the bowel will contain variable amounts of solid, liquid and gaseous constituents. CT imaging frequently identifies the cause of obstruction.

 KEY POINTS

- Dilatation of the colon >6 cm is abnormal (as is caecal dilatation >9 cm).
- An abdominal radiograph may demonstrate the level of large bowel obstruction but cannot reliably differentiate mechanical obstruction from pseudo-obstruction.

History

A 74-year-old man with a 40-year history of smoking attends his general practitioner (GP). He has been coughing up blood-stained sputum over the past 2 months and has also noted some weight loss. Over the past 48 hours he has noticed increasing shortness of breath and some discomfort in the left side of his chest.

Examination

A full blood count and urea and electrolytes are normal. He is referred for a chest radiograph (Figure 53.1) and, based on the results of the chest X-ray, he is referred to hospital for a computed tomography (CT) scan (Figure 53.2).

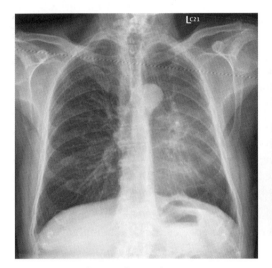

Figure 53.1 Chest radiograph.

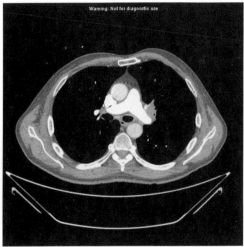

Figure 53.2 Axial enhanced CT scan.

Questions

- What does the chest radiograph show?
- Why can you not see the left heart border?
- Is the left hilum of normal appearance?
- What does the CT scan show?

ANSWER 53

In the chest radiograph (Figure 53.1) there is diffuse haziness over the left hemithorax which is caused by the collapse (atelectasis) of the left upper lobe which lies as a thin curtain over the remaining inflated left lower lobe. There is a left hilar mass, which is the likely cause for the lobar collapse. On the axial enhanced CT image (Figure 53.2) an obstructing left hilar mass is seen along with an adjacent parenchymal mass.

It is important to be aware that the left upper lobe does not collapse in the same manner as the right upper lobe. This is due to anatomy as there is no middle lobe on the left. The equivalent of the right middle lobe on the left is the lingula segment of the left upper lobe.

Plain film signs of left upper lobe collapse include: an area of increased opacity in the left upper lobe with a poorly defined margin on posterior–anterior (PA) radiograph, the left hilum may be elevated and an increase in lung density which may be almost imperceptible on the PA view. The aortic knob and upper left cardiac shadow may be obliterated and there may be a lucent stripe between the medial edge of the collapsed segment and the aortic arch (where the lower lobe has been pulled up by the collapsed lung – the Luftsichel sign). Unlike right upper lobe collapse, there is no sharply defined border and the abnormal increase in lung density merges into the normal lung inferiorly.

Lobar collapse is divided physiologically into obstructive and non-obstructive causes. Obstructive atelectasis is the most common form and results from reabsorption of gas from the alveoli when communication between the alveoli and the trachea is obstructed. The obstruction can occur at the level of the larger or smaller bronchus. Common causes of obstructive atelectasis include foreign body, tumour and mucous plugging.

Non-obstructive atelectasis can be caused by loss of contact between the parietal and visceral pleurae, compression, loss of surfactant and replacement of parenchymal tissue by scarring or infiltrative disease.

Collapse and consolidation can occur independently or together. Collapse can be partial or complete. Consolidation alone is not associated with a reduction in volume of the affected lung. It is often not clear to what extent the appearance is due to collapse or consolidation or both. If a lobe is only partially collapsed and there is no accompanying consolidation, there may be no increase in opacity. In cases of pure collapse, only when the collapse is virtually complete will there be a significant increase in density of the affected lung.

 KEY POINTS

- Left upper lobe collapse may be a subtle finding on chest radiograph.
- In the context of the clinical history, given this is highly suspicious for collapse secondary to an obstructing bronchogenic malignancy further imaging with CT should be performed for further evaluation.

History

A 35-year-old man who is otherwise fit and well with no previous medical history attends his general practitioner (GP) with an 18-month history of a soft swelling over his lumbar spine. The lump has not changed in size over the last year. He has noticed it incidentally and it has not been uncomfortable. No other lumps have been noted. He is concerned regarding its aesthetic appearance and wants to get it checked.

Examination

On examination the lump was soft, fluctuant, not fixed to underlying tissues and there was no overlying skin changes. It was a solitary lesion. There was no pulsatility. It did not transilluminate. The GP suspected a benign lesion but wanted correlation with ultrasound (Figures 54.1 and 54.2).

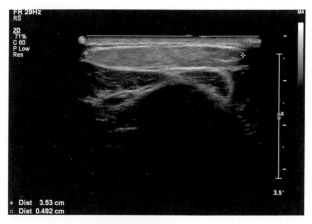

Figure 54.1 Ultrasound.

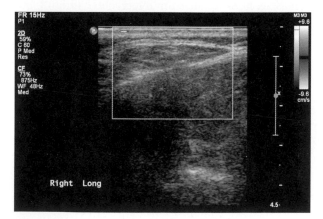

Figure 54.2 Ultrasound with colour Doppler.

Question

- What do you think is the most likely diagnosis?
- How would you describe the ultrasound findings?

ANSWER 54

Figure 54.1 is an ultrasound image demonstrating an ovoid hypoechoic subcutaneous lesion parallel to the skin with no evidence of invasion into deeper structures. There are septations seen internally. Sonographic features are consistent with a lipoma. The same lesion with colour Doppler settings applied (Figure 54.2) shows that the lesion is avascular, consistent with a lipoma.

Lipomas are the most common benign mesenchymal tumour. These slow-growing, benign fatty tumours form soft, lobulated masses enclosed by a thin, fibrous capsule. Although it has been suggested that lipomas may rarely undergo sarcomatous (malignant) change, this has never been convincingly proven. The majority of lipomas encountered by clinicians are subcutaneous in location. Lipomas typically develop as discrete rubbery masses in the subcutaneous tissues of the trunk and proximal extremities. Occasionally they may be found in other locations, for example, intramuscular, retroperitoneal and gastrointestinal.

Patients usually give a history of a slowly growing lesion present for years and usually do not complain of pain or discomfort. Painful lipomas are the hallmark of a rare condition called Dercum's disease (adiposis dolorosa).

In the subcutaneous location, the primary differential diagnosis is a sebaceous cyst or an abscess. Sebaceous cysts are also rounded and subcutaneous. They can be differentiated from lipomas by their characteristic central punctum and the surrounding induration. Treatment requires removal of a small ellipse of overlying skin to avoid entering the cyst. Abscesses typically have overlying induration and erythema. In these cases, incision and drainage is the appropriate management.

On ultrasound, subcutaneous lipomas are usually seen as well-defined, compressible, elliptical masses with the longest diameter parallel to the skin surface. They demonstrate multiple echogenic lines parallel to the skin surface with no evidence of posterior enhancement or attenuation and no flow on colour Doppler sonography (as seen in Figure 54.2). Compared with adjacent muscle, most lipomas are hyperechoic (bright), but some may be isoechoic or hypoechoic (dark).

CT scanning is principally indicated for distinguishing between lipomas and liposarcomas.

 KEY POINTS

- Subcutaneous lipomas are common, slow-growing, benign soft tissue tumours.
- Sonographically they are usually seen as well-defined, avascular, compressible, elliptical masses with the longest diameter parallel to the skin surface.

History

A 61-year-old man presents to hospital with generalized abdominal distension and bloating over the previous 3 weeks. This has become increasingly uncomfortable. He also notes feeling tired and lethargic.

Examination

Upon examination his observations are all within normal limits. His chest is clear but the abdomen is markedly distended. Upon percussing the abdomen there is dullness which moves depending on the position of the patient (shifting dullness). Bowel sounds are present but reduced. Rectal examination reveals an empty rectum.

His haemoglobin is reduced at 9.6 g/dL with evidence of a microcytic anaemia. Otherwise his blood biochemisty, liver function test and inflammatory markers are normal.

An ultrasound was performed in the first instance (Figure 55.1) and on the basis of this a computed tomography (CT) was done (Figure 55.2).

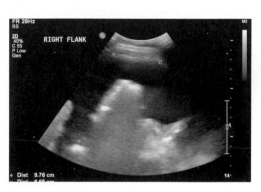

Figure 55.1 Ultrasound.

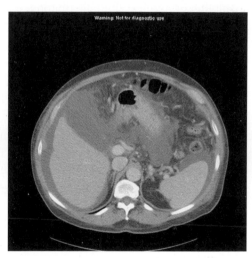

Figure 55.2 CT scan.

Questions

- What do the ultrasound image and the CT image demonstrate?
- What are the potential causes that could give rise to this?

ANSWER 55

The ultrasound image in Figure 55.1 demonstrates a large, anechoic (in other words, no echoes or solid component) fluid collection within the abdomen. The edge of the liver is seen in the bottom left of the image and collapsed loops of bowel are seen inferiorly and to the right. The ultrasound image has been acquired with the probe held in a longitudinal orientation in the subphrenic region.

The axial contrast enhanced CT image in Figure 55.2 confirms a large volume of fluid around the inferior margin of the liver, the spleen and within the upper abdomen.

Ascites describes the condition of pathological collection of fluid within the abdominal cavity and there is a wide differential of both transudative and exudative causes.

Uncomplicated (in other words non-infected, inflammatory or malignant) ascites appears as a homogeneous, freely mobile, anechoic collection in the peritoneal cavity demonstrating acoustic enhancement. Free ascites does not displace organs but typically distributes itself between them, conforming to organ margins.

Features suggesting complicated ascites include fine or coarse internal echoes, septation, loculation or atypical fluid distribution, matting/clumping of bowel loops and thickening of interfaces between the fluid and adjacent structures.

Traces of fluid usually collect in the posterior subhepatic space (Morrison's pouch) and around the liver as a sonolucent (dark on ultrasound) band. Fluid also often localizes in the pouch of Douglas (recto-uterine pouch). Where there is a large volume of ascites, the small bowel loops have a characteristic appearance on ultrasound as they hang from a vertically floating mesentery.

Ascites is also usually demonstrated well on CT scanning. CT may also demonstrate the aetiology including features suggestive of neoplasia such as hepatic, splenic or adrenal lesions, lymphadenopathy or masses arising from the bowel, ovary or pancreas.

This patient was found to have a gastrointestinal stromal tumour as the cause of his ascites.

 KEY POINTS

- Ultrasound and CT are both sensitive to small volumes of ascites and may demonstrate the aetiology.

History

A 55-year-old woman presents to her general practitioner (GP) with several weeks of pain in the left hand. She remembers tripping in the garden and landing on her left outstretched hand previously but had not attended the accident and emergency department, as she did not feel she had sustained a fracture.

She is otherwise fit and well. Her symptoms include pain (which she describes as 'burning' type), tenderness and swelling in the left hand.

Examination

On examination there is wasting of the intrinsic muscles of the hand associated with evidence of sweating, warmth and flushed, shiny skin. There was evidence of hyperaesthesia, hyperalgesia and allodynia. There was no evidence of synovitis or deformity, however. The GP decided to refer the patient to her local hospital for an X-ray (Figures 56.1a,b).

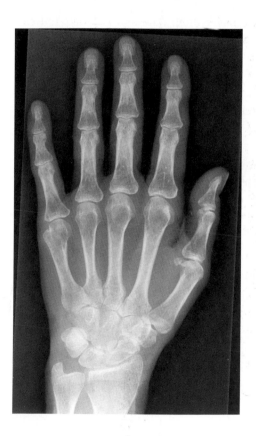 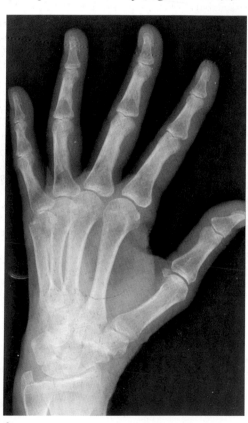

(b)

Figure 56.1 (a) Posterior–anterior (PA) and (b) oblique views.

Question

• What abnormality do you notice on these hand radiographs?

There is diffuse reduction in radiological bone density (increased radiolucency) in a predominantly periarticular distribution around the joints of the hand. There is, however, no associated evidence of joint erosions or destruction and no focal destructive cortical bony lesion or periosteal reaction is seen. Features are consistent with a regional periarticular osteopaenia.

Osteopaenia refers to reduced bone mineral density and, radiologically, to increased radiolucency of bone. The most common cause by far of osteopaenia is osteoporosis, however, there are multiple aetiologies so the finding of radiolucent bone does not make this an automatic diagnosis. One should search for other more specific clues to the exact underlying disorder and more specific radiographic clues to their diagnosis.

Osteopaenia can be difficult to diagnose accurately on plain radiographs which are frequently insensitive to changes in bone mineral. Approximately 30–50 per cent of the bone mass must be lost before it can be detected on a plain film.

Osteopaenia may be diffuse or regional and the differential diagnosis is broad and can be vascular, drug-induced, toxic, endocrine/metabolic, congenital or idiopathic. Causes of regional osteoporosis include immobilization with disuse and regional sympathetic dystrophy syndrome (RSDS).

In the hand radiographs seen in Figures 56.1, the joint spaces are generally preserved with no destructive changes. The history, examination and imaging features suggested regional osteoporosis secondary to RSDS.

The exact mechanism of how RSDS develops is poorly understood. Theories include irritation and abnormal excitation of nervous tissue, leading to abnormal impulses along nerves that affect blood vessels and skin. A variety of events can trigger the condition, including trauma, surgery, heart disease, degenerative arthritis of the neck, stroke or other brain diseases, nerve irritation by entrapment (such as carpal tunnel syndrome), shoulder problems, breast cancer, and drugs for tuberculosis and barbiturates. The incidence after fractures and contusions ranges from 10 to 30 per cent. In this case the patient had sustained trauma in the absence of a fracture. While some cases are associated with an identifiable nerve injury, many are not and there is no associated event in a third of patients. The upper extremities are more likely to be involved than the lower.

 KEY POINTS

- Osteopaenia refers to increased radiolucency of bone. The most common cause by far of osteopaenia is osteoporosis.
- Osteopaenia can be diffuse or localized. Secondary clues should be sought to identify the aetiology.

History

A 65-year-old retired construction worker attends his general practitioner (GP) with a cough. The cough was non-productive and he denied feeling significantly short of breath. He also denied fevers and weight loss. He was a non-smoker and had been otherwise well aside from taking a thiazide diuretic for hypertension, which was well controlled. He had only a history of hernia repair and appendicectomy many years previously. In his occupational history, he had retired from construction work aged 50 and had worked in an administrative role for the last 15 years.

Examination

On examination he looked well. There was good air entry and chest expansion bilaterally, breath sounds were vesicular and there were no added sounds.

A routine chest radiograph was performed (Figure 57.1). Upon reviewing the radiograph the GP requested a computed tomography (CT) scan of the thorax (Figure 57.2).

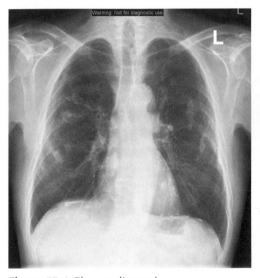

Figure 57.1 Chest radiograph.

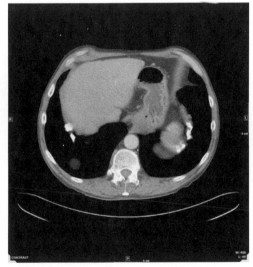

Figure 57.2 CT scan of thorax.

Questions

- What do the chest radiograph and the CT scan demonstrate?
- What may cause this appearance?

The chest radiograph in Figure 57.1 demonstrates multiple bilateral radio-opaque pleural plaques consistent with previous exposure to asbestos. This is confirmed on CT in Figure 57.2 where calcified pleural plaques are seen along the diaphragmatic pleura.

Pleural plaques are deposits of hyalinized collagen fibres in the parietal pleura. They are indicative of asbestos exposure and typically become visible after a latency period of 10–20 or more years after the inhalation of asbestos fibres. Asbestos is a naturally occurring fibrous silicate that was widely used in the past for a range of commercial applications including shipbuilding, construction, textile and insulation industries.

In addition to benign pleural plaques, however, there is also a spectrum of more significant asbestos-related thoracic diseases including benign pleural effusion, diffuse pleural thickening, rounded atelectasis, asbestosis (i.e. lung fibrosis), mesothelioma and lung cancer. Plaques may occur in isolation as in this case or in association with lung parenchymal disease.

Pleural plaques are usually multiple, bilateral and often relatively symmetrical and are located in the mid portion of the chest wall between the seventh and tenth ribs, following rib contours, or adjacent to the aponeurotic portion of the diaphragm (as seen on the CT). Visceral pleura, lung apices and costophrenic angles are usually spared.

On chest radiographs, the prevalence of calcification in pleural plaques is reported to be around 15 per cent, however CT is far more sensitive with sensitivity around 50 per cent. In profile, calcified plaques appear as opaque lines that lie parallel to the chest wall, mediastinum, pericardium and diaphragm. Viewed en face, calcified plaques are seen as irregular and heterogeneous densities. The presence of bilateral, superior diaphragmatic surface calcifications with spared costophrenic angles is virtually pathognomonic for asbestos-related pleural disease. Isolated plaques and diffuse pleural thickening may also seen in tuberculosis, trauma and haemothorax.

CT scanning is often used in the evaluation of pleural disease. Plaques appear as discrete, well-defined areas of localized pleural thickening which are usually multiple, bilateral and located adjacent to rigid structures, such as the ribs, mid portion of the chest, aponeurotic portion of the diaphragm, mediastinum and paravertebral regions. Lung apices and costophrenic angles typically are spared. Rarely, the visceral pleura within fissures may be involved, or plaques may be pedunculated.

CT scanning (in particular, high-resolution CT) allows demonstration of interstitial infiltrates and fibrosis, and may be helpful in diagnosing early stages of asbestosis. It also is useful in delineation of pleural or pleura-based abnormalities (for example, effusion, thickening, plaque, malignant mesothelioma, rounded atelectasis) and in evaluation of a parenchymal density that is suggestive of bronchogenic carcinoma.

In this case, the CT failed to show any further significant sequelae of asbestos exposure and the patient recovered with a short course of antibiotics. In the absence of any other sign of asbestos-related disease, isolated pleural plaques alone do not require further follow-up or investigation.

 KEY POINTS

- Latency time for development of pleural plaques is usually around 20 years.
- Most patients who have asbestos-related pleural plaques are asymptomatic. The chest radiograph plays an important role in detection of asbestos-related pleural and parenchymal abnormalities and assessment of progression of disease.
- High-resolution CT is superior to the radiograph in detection of pleural plaques and is more sensitive and specific for the diagnosis of asbestos-related pleural disease.

History

A 38-year-old man attends the accident and emergency department with a 48-hour history of cramping abdominal pain associated with nausea and vomiting. He felt his abdomen was 'blown up' and mentioned no longer being able to pass flatus. He was also sweating and thirsty.

Five years previously he had a prolonged admission following a perforated appendix for which he had his appendix removed and an associated abscess drained. He had remained well ever since, took no medications and had no allergies.

Examination

On examination his pulse was 104/minute, in sinus rhythm. His mucous membranes were dry. His abdomen was distended. He complained of generalized tenderness but there was no rebound or guarding. The bowel sounds were prominent and tympanic. Per rectal exam demonstrated an empty rectum.

His blood results demonstrated normal inflammatory markers. His biochemistry revealed a urea of 8.4 mmol/L but creatinine within the normal range.

An erect chest radiograph was performed which did not demonstrate any free subdiaphragmatic gas, but the abdominal radiograph (Figure 58.1) was abnormal. In light of this and following surgical review, a computed tomography (CT) scan was performed (Figure 58.2).

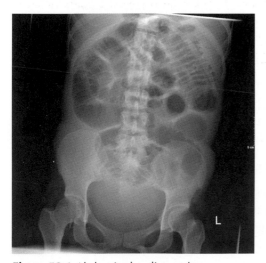

Figure 58.1 Abdominal radiograph.

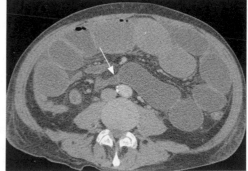

Figure 58.2 CT scan.

Questions

- What abnormality is seen on the plain abdominal radiograph (Figure 58.1)?
- What does the CT show (Figure 58.2)?
- What does the arrow point to?

The radiograph of the abdomen in Figure 58.1 demonstrates multiple abnormally distended loops of small bowel. No surgical clips are seen. The large bowel is collapsed. It is possible to determine that this is small bowel dilatation, by the central location, calibre and the presence of valvulae conniventes (as opposed to the peripheral location, wider calibre and haustral folds of the large bowel). There is no evidence of pneumoperitoneum to suggest perforation. The axial CT in Figure 58.2 confirms dilated loops of fluid-filled small bowel.

A small bowel obstruction is caused by a variety of pathologic processes but essentially is due to mechanical obstruction to the passage of the bowel contents somewhere in the small bowel. The bowel proximal to the point of obstruction dilates with swallowed air and secreted fluid. Vomiting may release some of the proximal bowel contents and reduce the amount of proximal dilation. Bowel distal to the point of obstruction (i.e. colon and distal small bowel) empties and collapses over time

The leading cause in developed countries is postoperative adhesions (60 per cent). Postoperative adhesions can be the cause of acute obstruction within weeks of surgery or present as chronic obstruction years later as in this case.

The second most common identified cause of small bowel obstruction is an incarcerated groin hernia. Other aetiologies include malignant tumor (20 per cent), other hernias (10 per cent), inflammatory bowel disease (5 per cent), volvulus (3 per cent) and other causes (2 per cent).

Small bowel obstructions can be partial or complete. They may also be simple or strangulated. Strangulated obstructions are surgical emergencies. If not diagnosed and properly treated, vascular compromise can lead to bowel ischaemia, morbidity and mortality.

Plain radiographs are the primary imaging modality with the sensitivity reported as approximately 75 per cent. Assessment should be made for surgical clips (which may suggest adhesions as a cause), the hernial orifices (for incarcerated hernia) or aerobilia/calcific densities (possible gallstone ileus). Small bowel dilatation greater than 2.5–3 cm (especially if there is evidence of air–fluid levels) indicates small bowel obstruction.

CT scanning is useful in distinguishing extrinsic causes, for example adhesions and hernias, from intrinsic causes, such as neoplasms or Crohn's disease. A transition point may be identified localizing any focal adhesions, as seen on the axial CT image in Figure 58.2 (arrow), which cannot be appreciated on plain films. The patient in this case probably developed adhesions as a consequence of the surgery for his perforated appendix and abscess drainage.

CT should be considered where the patient has fever, tachycardia and localized abdominal pain with raised inflammatory markers. CT may demonstrate abscesses, inflammatory processes, extraluminal pathology resulting in obstruction, tumours or mesenteric ischaemia. It also allows discrimination between ileus and mechanical small bowel in postoperative patients.

KEY POINTS

- In cases of small bowel obstruction, plain radiographs are the primary imaging modality and assessment should be made for surgical clips (which may suggest adhesions), hernial orifices (for incarcerated hernia) or aerobilia/calcific densities (possible gallstone ileus).
- CT scanning is useful in distinguishing the aetiology and also allows discrimination between ileus and mechanical small bowel in postoperative patients.

History

A 52-year-old man with a history of alcoholism and hepatitis C is admitted to intensive care with torrential haematemesis. He requires the transfusion of 10 units of blood, clotting factor and platelets over 36 hours. Upper gastrointestinal endoscopy reveals large clots seen within the stomach with an associated bleeding point as a result of varices.

Examination

The patient is tachycardic with a pulse rate of 108/minute and tachypnoeic at 22/minute. His blood pressure has been maintained within normal limits with replacement of blood and colloids. Despite best efforts, however, the endoscopist is unable to halt the gastric bleeding and a computed tomography (CT) scan is therefore performed to assess for any potential point of arterial embolization (Figure 59.1a,b).

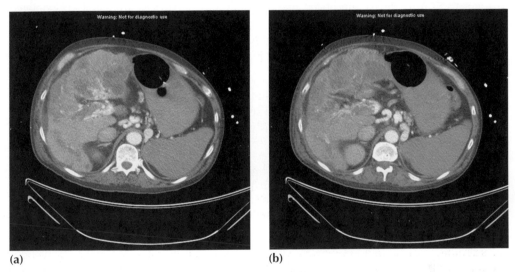

(a)   (b)

Figure 59.1 Two axial contrast-enhanced CT images.

Question

- What abnormalities do the two axial contrast-enhanced CT images in Figure 59.1a,b demonstrate?

ANSWER 59

The axial contrast-enhanced CT images in Figure 59.1 are taken at two levels through the upper abdomen and demonstrate the presence of enhancing serpigenous veins adjacent to the stomach consistent with gastric varices as a consequence of liver cirrhosis (irregular liver contour, patchy low attenuation and enhancement) and portal venous thrombosis (filling defect within the portal vein), which are also seen.

Gastric varices are dilated submucosal veins in the stomach, which are most frequently found in patients with portal hypertension and resulting elevated portal venous pressure, which may be a complication of cirrhosis. In this example, the portal vein itself is thrombosed.

Gastric variceal bleeding is often profuse, has a high rate of recurrence and is associated with decreased survival. Bleeding varices represent a potentially life-threatening cause of haematemesis.

In the setting of cirrhosis and portal hypertension, gastric varices are usually associated with oesophageal varices. Isolated gastric varices may also be found in patients with splenic venous thrombosis as blood is shunted via the short gastric veins, which drain the fundus of the stomach flow. For example, this may be a complication of acute pancreatitis or pancreatic malignancy.

Patients with bleeding gastric varices in addition to presenting with haematemesis, may exhibit melaena or frank rectal bleeding. The bleeding may be brisk, and patients may soon develop haemorrhagic shock, with this patient clinically demonstrating features of grade 2 shock.

Gastric varices are seen on CT (Figure 59.1) as characteristically multiple lobulated, serpentine masses. It is possible for varices to present as a polypoid mass in the fundus. They may also be seen on ultrasound of the upper abdomen or on upper gastrointestinal barium series (although they may be obscured by overlying gastric rugae).

On this occasion, no focal bleeding point was identified as suitable for embolization.

 KEY POINTS

- CT or ultrasound may demonstrate evidence of liver cirrhosis, portal hypertension and ascites in addition to the varices themselves.

CASE 60: AN INCIDENTAL FINDING ON CHEST RADIOGRAPH

History
A previously fit and well 16-year-old boy attends his general practitioner (GP) with a 2-week history of a cough. He noted a small amount of clear sputum but the cough had been generally non-productive and there had been no blood expectorated. He had noted feeling generally feverish. He had been previously fit and well.

Examination
On examination he demonstrates evidence of an upper tract respiratory infection. He was afebrile, with a respiratory rate of 20/minute and a heart rate of 80/minute. On respiratory examination there is equal lung expansion with good air entry bilaterally. Breath sounds were vesicular with no added sounds. Investigations showed a normal white cell count and a slightly elevated C-reactive protein of 20 mg/L. Blood biochemistry was normal. The GP referred him to his local hospital for a chest radiograph (Figures 60.1 and 60.2).

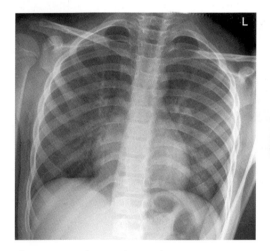

Figure 60.1 Chest radiograph

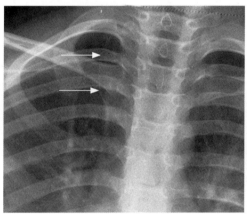

Figure 60.2 Chest radiograph

Questions
- What do you observe about the chest radiograph (Figure 60.1)?
- What do the arrows identify (Figure 60.2)?
- What is the significance of this finding?

ANSWER 60

Figure 60.1 shows a normal heart size and mediastinal contour with no focal collapse, consolidation or active pulmonary lesion. The pleural spaces are clear. Incidental note is made of an azygos fissure.

The arrows in Figure 60.2 identify an azygos fissure (azygos lobe), which is a small accessory lobe sometimes found on the upper part of the right lung, separated from the rest of the upper lobe by a deep groove lodging the azygos vein, of little clinical significance.

The azygos lobe appears commencing in a 'teardrop' shape approximately at around the level of T5 to the right of the midline as a pale line curving outward and upward, then back in to meet the root of the neck. The line is the infolding of the pleura.

Abnormal fissures and lobes of the lungs are common and usually insignificant. A lobe related to the azygos vein appears in the right lung in about 1–2 per cent of people. It develops when the apical bronchus grows superiorly and medial to the arch of the azygos vein (instead of lateral to it). As a consequence, the azygos vein comes to lie at the bottom of a deep fissure in the superior lobe of the right lung.

In this patient, no focal active lung pathology was identified. Incidental note was made of the azygos lobe. No further investigation or treatment is required.

 KEY POINTS

- An azygos lobe is frequently an incidental finding on chest radiograph and usually has no clinical significance.

History

A 64-year-old man is admitted to intensive care following a coronary artery bypass graft and aortic valve replacement. The procedure was uncomplicated, but post-operatively he is slow to regain his appetite and a nasogastric tube is placed on intensive care for enteral feeding. The nurse uses litmus paper to test the acidity of the aspirates and is concerned. Simultaneously, the patient shortly afterwards begins to become dyspnoeic and is making gagging reflexes.

Examination

His saturations drop to 82–86 per cent on 8L of oxygen. His blood pressure and heart rate remain within normal limits. A chest radiograph is performed urgently (Figure 61.1).

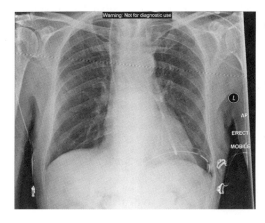

Figure 61.1 Chest radiograph.

Questions

- What abnormality do you note on the chest radiograph in Figure 61.1?
- What other findings are there on the image?
- What has changed in Figure 61.2?
- What abnormality does Figure 61.3 show (taken from a different paediatric patient)?

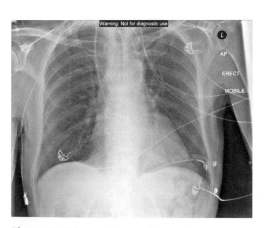

Figure 61.2 Later chest radiograph.

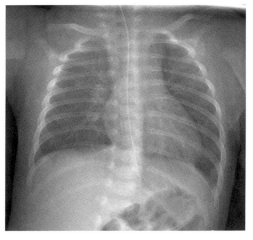

Figure 61.3 Chest radiograph from a different (paediatric) patient.

The chest radiograph in Figure 61.1 shows that the nasogastric (NG) tube has been passed down the left main bronchus. This is unusual as the (less acute) angle of the right main bronchus is usually more favourable. There is a right internal jugular catheter which is appropriately placed with its tip projected over the superior vena cava/right atrium. A left intercostal chest drain is seen. Sternal wires are noted. Figure 61.2 demonstrates the appropriately repositioned NG tube extending below the diaphragm. Figure 61.3 demonstrates an NG tube in a different (paediatric) patient, which lies within the distal oesophagus and should be advanced into the stomach.

Chest radiographs for NG tube position are common. The NG tube is usually inserted either for providing enteral nutrition, administration of drugs or for gastric drainage. Nasogastric feeding is a common practice in all age groups. There is a risk that the NG feeding tube can be misplaced into the lungs during insertion (as in Figure 61.1) or may move out of the stomach at a later stage (Figure 61.3).

In the past, various methods have been used to determine the position of NG feeding tubes. These included:

- auscultation of air insufflated through the feeding tube (listening for a 'whoosh');
- testing acidity or alkalinity of the aspirate using litmus paper;
- looking for bubbling at the end of the NG tube;
- the appearance of the feeding tube aspirate.

Current recommendations, however, suggest that these measures are not reliable and therefore should not be used to detect the position of NG tubes.

The position of the tip of the NGT is assessed frequently in the first instance by drawing back gastric contents and testing with pH paper. If there is any concern then radiographic confirmation of NG tube position is performed.

Indeed current guidelines suggest:

- measuring the pH of the aspirate using pH indicator strips;
- use of radiography.

The most accurate method for confirming the correct position of an NG feeding tube is radiography. The aim of radiography is to positively confirm that the NG tube is within the gastrointestinal tract (within the stomach).

Sometimes longer nasojejunal (NJ) tubes are used. The objective is to place the tip of the tube past the pylorus, through the duodenum and beyond the duodenal–jejunal flexure into the jejunum. In doing so, this bypasses the regulatory function of the pylorus and delivers nutrition or therapeutic agents directly into the jejunum.

The importance of establishing the position of the NG tube cannot be understated. A patient who is fed or administered drugs via a malpositioned NG tube, such as that in Figure 61.1, can deteriorate significantly and it may even lead to iatrogenic death.

 KEY POINTS

- Current guidelines for appropriate placement of NG tubes include measuring the pH of the aspirate using pH indicator strips and use of chest radiography to ensure the tip of the tube is sited appropriately.

History

A 24-year-old man presents to the accident and emergency department with vomiting and abdominal pain that has been worsening over the last 24 hours. He describes initially feeling unwell with mild fever and central abdominal discomfort that has slowly focused into the right iliac fossa. He has not been exposed to other people with similar symptoms and although he has bought and eaten freshly prepared food, none of his friends have has similar symptoms. He has no significant medical history.

Examination

His temperature is 37.8°C but his observations are otherwise normal. His chest and heart sounds are normal. On abdominal examination there is mild distension and tenderness over the right iliac fossa but no rebound tenderness. Bowel sounds are reduced.

You arrange an abdominal radiograph (Figure 62.1) and an ultrasound (Figure 62.2), among other tests.

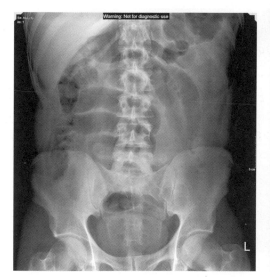

Figure 62.1 Abdominal radiograph.

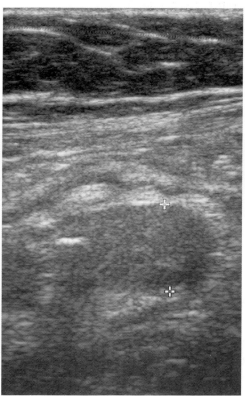

Figure 62.2 Ultrasound image of the right iliac fossa.

Questions

- What do the investigations show?
- What differential diagnoses could give these appearances?
- What else would you like to know?
- Would you do more imaging?

The abdominal radiograph (Figure 62.1) shows dilated lucent loops of small bowel, likely to be partially gas filled in the upper abdomen. The distal small bowel is not seen, probably fluid filled and no comment about dilatation can be made. The large bowel gas pattern is not abnormal. The appearance could indicate a small bowel ileus or obstruction, although a transition point to indicate a mechanical obstruction is not seen.

The ultrasound of the right iliac fossa (Figure 62.2) shows a tubular structure measuring 1.3 cm containing a calcification that blocks the ultrasound beam and casts a shadow that may represent a dilated appendix (>6 mm diameter). The upper abdomen is normal. The bladder appears normal. No significant free fluid is seen.

The differential diagnosis includes appendicitis, mesenteric adenitis (usually children), gastroenteritis, Crohn's disease, urinary tract infection and, in women, ovulation pain, ovarian cyst haemorrhage, torsion, ectopic pregnancy and pelvic inflammatory disease.

Appendicitis seems the most likely diagnosis, however tests should include urinalysis. In women, a pregnancy test should be done and it can be difficult to entirely rule out ovarian causes or pelvic inflammatory disease and a transvaginal ultrasound may be helpful although may not be acceptable in younger females. The diagnosis may end up being primarily clinical although a computed tomography (CT) may be done (as in this case due to the dilated small bowel) if it is considered that the additional information justifies the X-ray dose (Figure 62.3).

Appendicitis with small bowel dilatation is associated with a higher incidence of perforation of the appendix.

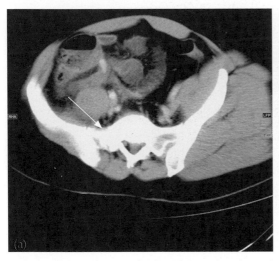 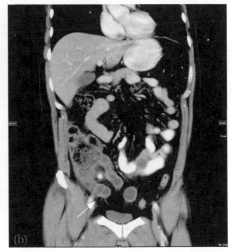

Figure 62.3 (a) Oblique axial and (b) coronal CT slices of the abdomen and pelvis showing a large appendicolith (present in 25 per cent on CT) within the dilated appendix (white arrows) with surrounding inflammatory change of the fat and caecal pole.

🔧 **KEY POINTS**

- Ultrasound may occasionally diagnose appendicitis but may struggle to rule out many of the differential diagnoses.
- Ultrasound may be useful where there is reasonably high suspicion for appendicitis in children and young women where a CT scan may be avoided.

History

A 41-year-old woman is referred to the outpatient rheumatology clinic complaining of painful joints. The symptoms have been longstanding for 4 months and intermittently cause an achy pain in the finger joints of both hands. This is sometimes associated with joint swelling and causes stiffness, which is constant and not worse at any particular time of the day. She denies any stigmata of infection, weight loss or rash.

Approximately 5 years ago she was diagnosed with psoriasis for which she takes topical coal tar which controls her skin plaques well. She has no other relevant past medical history and does not take any other regular medication. She finds her job as a nursery school teacher very rewarding, but is finding her fine motor skill inhibited by joint stiffness when trying to help the children in arts and crafts lessons. She is a smoker of approximately 10 per week and drinks at weekends only. She is unmarried but lives with her boyfriend.

Examination reveals mildly swollen proximal interphalangeal joints bilaterally, which are tender and have slightly limited range of movement. Bloods are taken and a radiograph of both hands is ordered (Figure 63.1).

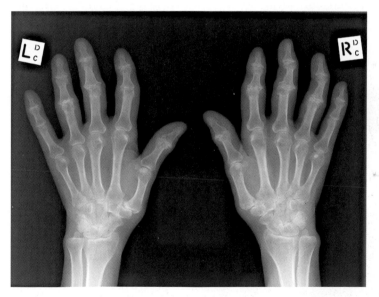

Figure 63.1 Anterior–posterior (AP) radiograph of both hands.

Questions

- What does the radiograph demonstrate?
- What is the main differential for these appearances?
- What are the extra-articular manifestations of rheumatoid arthritis?

ANSWER 63

Figure 63.1 is an AP radiograph of both hands in an adult female patient. Soft tissue swelling is seen involving the proximal interphalangeal joints (PIPJs). There is a symmetrical distal small joint polyarthropathy. This predominantly involves the second, third and fourth PIPJs of both hands with less marked involvement of the first interphalangeal joints and the distal interphalangeal joints (DIPJs). The involved joints demonstrate loss of normal cartilage and reduced joint space with marginal juxta-articular erosions. These are poorly demarcated and partially obscured with overlying new bone formation, suggesting periostitis, and are termed 'proliferative erosions'. The PIPJ articular surfaces are irregular, but there is no subperiosteal osteoporosis or articular erosive changes seen to suggest a 'pencil in cup' appearance.

Bone density is preserved throughout and there is no bony ankylosis. The metacarpophalangeal joints are preserved, but there is mild radiocarpal and carpometacarpal joint space narrowing in keeping with degenerative change. These appearances are characteristic of a seronegative spondyloarthropathy most likely related to psoriasis, however a diagnosis of rheumatoid arthritis needs to be excluded.

Psoriasis is a chronic inflammatory skin condition, which can affect people at any age. It is characterized by the presence of red skin plaques that are raised from the skin and is often capped by silvery scales, associated with nail changes. It has a predilection for extensor sites and is most commonly identified at the elbow and knee joints. There are well-documented extracutaneous manifestations with arthropathy affecting 5 per cent of psoriatic suffers and sometimes preceding the skin plaques by many years. There five radiological subtypes of psoriatic arthropathy:[1,2]

- symmetrical polyarthritis of the interphalangeal joints;
- seronegative polyarthritis mimicking rheumatoid arthritis;
- monoarthritis or asymmetrical oligoarthritis;
- spondyloarthritis mimicking ankylosing spondylitis;
- arthritis mutilans – a severe form of arthritis with marked deformity and joint destruction.

In contrast, Figure 63.2 is a characteristic plain radiograph of both hands in a patient with longstanding rheumatoid arthritis. There is marked erosive change and fusion

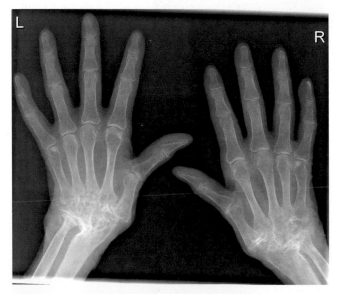

Figure 63.2 Plain radiograph of both hands in a patient with longstanding rheumatoid arthritis.

related to the carpal bones bilaterally with erosive changes also seen related to the distal radius and ulna. Bone density is generally reduced and there is bony ankylosis of the carpometacarpal joints. The PIPJs and DIPJs are preserved throughout.

Rheumatoid arthritis is an immunologically mediated multisystem collagen vascular disease of unknown aetiology. Treatment in the acute setting of joint involvement is similar to that of psoriasis, but long-term treatment is complicated, often involving a delicate balance of disease modifying drugs (DMARDs) requiring regular clinical follow-up and blood tests. Being a multisystem disorder, rheumatoid arthritis can affect the patient in many ways outside of joint involvement. These include:

- systemic illness – fever, malaise and weight loss;
- vasculitis – predominantly affecting small vessels, the disease can mimic polyarteritis nodosa causing peripheral neuropathy;
- skin nodules – firm and tender skin nodules occur along tendon sheaths;
- respiratory disorders – lung nodularity with cavitation can be seen, with concomitant pulmonary fibrosis and pleural effusion;
- cardiovascular disorders – pericarditis, pericardial effusion and myositis are recognized;
- Felty's syndrome – massive splenomegaly, often with neutropenia.

 KEY POINTS

- Joint disease can precede the cutaneous manifestations of psoriasis by several years.
- Classically, psoriasis is associated with a symmetrical distal polyarthropathy of the interphalangeal joints.
- Rheumatoid arthritis predominantly affects the distal radius and proximal joints of the hand bilaterally.

References

1. Chapman, S. and Nakielny, R. *Aids to Radiological Differential Diagnosis*, 4th edn. Philadelphia: W.B. Saunders.
2. Jacobson, J.A., Girish, G., Jiang, Y. and Resnick, D. (2008) Radiographic evaluation of arthritis: inflammatory conditions. *Radiology* 248: 378–89.

History

A 38-year-old sports teacher was brought to the accident and emergency department by ambulance. He had been found unconscious in his office by another member of staff at the end of the afternoon. There was no sign of assault and the accompanying member of staff remembers seeing the sports teacher at lunch where they laughed together at something that had occurred that morning.

The sports teacher had taken his first class to the cricket nets for catching and batting practice. During the session a batsman had driven the ball hard, accidentally hitting the teacher on the left side of the head. Pupils near by heard a 'crack' but the sports teacher did not lose consciousness and carried on with the lesson. He did report at lunchtime feeling a little drowsy but had only administrative duties in the afternoon. On her way home, another teacher checked on the sports teacher to find him unrousable in his office and she raised the alarm.

Examination

Ambulance paramedics urgently brought the sports teacher to the accident and emergency department. Glasgow Coma Scale score (GCS) on arrival was 7 (motor 4, eyes 2, speech 1). He had been intubated in the resuscitation room to protect his airway, and a cranial computed tomography (CT) scan was performed before admission to intensive care (Figure 64.1).

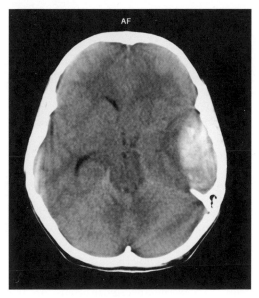

Figure 64.1 Axial cranial CT scan.

Questions

* What are the CT scan findings?
* What is the diagnosis?

ANSWER 64

Figure 64.1 shows a single slice of a cranial CT scan taken at the level of the caudate heads. There is asymmetry demonstrated with an area of increased density on the left side lying underneath the left temporal bone. This abnormality is more dense than adjacent brain parenchyma, but less dense than the skull bones in keeping with acute blood. It has a biconvex elliptical shape and is homogeneous in appearance. This collection of blood exerts mass effect on adjacent brain parenchyma with total effacement of the adjacent lateral ventricle and loss of normal left cerebral sulci. There is midline shift to the right of approximately 3 mm. The quadrageminal cistern is effaced but the right lateral ventricle remains of expected size.

The same image rewindowed to emphasize bony pathology (Figure 64.2) demonstrates a vertical fracture of the left temporal bone (arrow). There is some subcutaneous soft tissue thickening at this site, which corresponds to the site of impact of the cricket ball. This represents an acute extradural haemorrhage with mass effect compressing the brain within the skull.

Extradural haemorrhage is defined as a collection of blood within the space between the inner table of the skull and the dura mater of the meninges. Blood collects in the extradural space running along the inside of the skull. It is strongly associated with direct head trauma and skull fracture, with bony fragments lacerating the meningeal vessels (commonly middle meningeal). Depending on whether the lacerated vessels are arteries or veins, the rate of haematoma expansion dictates whether the patient presents hours or days after the incident. Common symptoms are of gradually increasing drowsiness, which can progress to coma as the haematoma has focal mass effect compressing the brain within the tight skull. Some patients can demonstrate a third nerve palsy or hemiparesis as a sign of cerebral herniation.

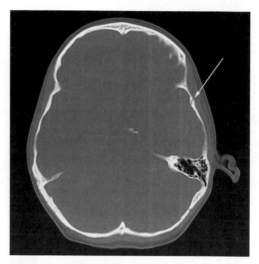

Figure 64.2 CT scan rewindowed to emphasize bony pathology.

An unenhanced cranial CT usually demonstrates an acute hyperdense collection of blood, but if a few days old, can have varied attenuation appearances. It is differentiated from other extra-axial collections by its shape. The expanding haematoma will have a biconvex elliptical shape as tracking blood is limited by the tethered cranial sutures. There may be a degree of mass effect, and image review with bone windows has a high sensitivity for resolving the underlying skull fracture. All patients will require urgent neurosurgical discussion and neurologically compromised patients will require urgent decompression and evacuation.

 KEY POINTS

- In an extradural haemorrhage, blood collects between the inner table of the skull and the dura mater.
- It classically presents with reduced conscious level several hours after a traumatic incident.
- A characteristic concave elliptical haematoma is seen on CT with tracking blood limited by cranial sutures.

CASE 65: A CHESTY INFANT

History

A 3-month-old boy was referred to the paediatric department by his general practitioner (GP) with respiratory problems. He has had a cough and runny nose for 2 days and has become progressively more chesty. He now has problems feeding, at least one episode of vomiting that may be cough related and dry nappies. Older siblings in the family also have coryzal symptoms. The patient was born 2 weeks prematurely with no significant neonatal problems. The mother is on treatment for asthma and there is no other significant medical or family history.

Examination

The initial examination showed a febrile infant with copious nasal secretions, conjunctivitis and noisy breathing (grunting and wheezing). There is tachypnoea (58 breaths per minute) with intercostal and subcostal retraction. On listening to the chest there are fine crackles and wheeze throughout. The rest of the examination is normal.

Over the next 24 hours, the patient did not improve on standard treatment and continuous positive airways pressure (CPAP) and eventually required intubation. At this point a chest radiograph (Figure 65.1) was done to check the lungs and position of the tube (an earlier radiograph had been unremarkable).

Six hours later, problems with ventilation developed and a further radiograph was done (Figure 65.2).

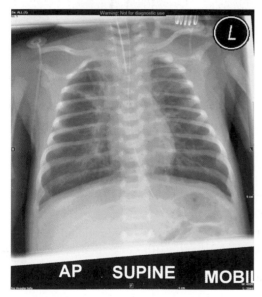
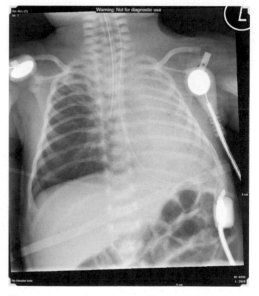

Figure 65.1 Anterior–posterior (AP) radiograph.

Figure 65.2 Later radiograph.

Questions

- What differentials are you considering?
- What does the first radiograph show?
- What complication has developed in the second radiograph and why?

ANSWER 65

Given the age and presentation, the most likely diagnosis is bronchiolitis although pneumonia and aspiration should also be considered. Undiagnosed congenital cardiac or lung disease and foreign body may need to be ruled out.

The first radiograph (Figure 65.1) shows hyperinflation with flattened diaphragm. The lung volumes are large due to air trapping rather than fortuitous timing of the radiograph. Coarsened lung markings that reflect patchy airspace and interstitial infiltrates are seen. There is also some thickening of the perihilar bronchial walls (cuffing). No focal consolidation, cardiac abnormality or foreign body is seen. The appearance is consistent with severe bronchiolitis, although similar appearances are also seen in atypical pneumonia and aspiration. The tip of the endotracheal (ET) tube is well above the carina and the tip of the nasogastric (NG) tube is below the diaphragm.

The second radiograph (Figure 65.2) shows a low ET tube in the right main bronchus resulting in left lung occlusion and collapse. Some compensatory hyperexpansion of the right lung across the midline is seen. The problem is remedied by withdrawing the tube tip (ideally to the level of the clavicles). Remember to comment on tubes and complications on every image.

The most common complication is bacterial coinfection. This was suspected in this patient's case and shown on a subsequent radiograph (Figure 65.3) that also showed re-expansion of the left lung.

Bronchiolitis is usually diagnosed clinically and a chest radiograph is only needed if the course of the illness is atypical or to rule out other causes or complications. The small airways become infected, resulting in narrowing and obstruction. The most common cause is the respiratory syncytial virus (RSV) and occasionally adenovirus and parainfluenza viruses. This may be confirmed by a nasopharyngeal aspirate. The illness can usually be managed at home, but 2–3 per cent of cases require admission to hospital of which 3–7 per cent require ventilation. Children

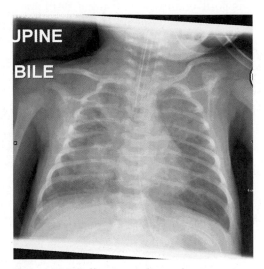

Figure 65.3 Follow-up radiograph.

with underlying cardiopulmonary disease, infants with a history of gestational age less than 34 weeks, infants younger than 6 weeks, and infants with congenital or acquired immunodeficiency are at high risk for severe RSV infection.

 KEY POINTS

- Bronchiolitis is largely diagnosed and managed without imaging.
- A chest radiograph is helpful to check for other causes and complications.
- The radiograph appearance of bronchiolitis is non-specific and may consist of hyperexpanded lungs only, although patchy infiltrates may also be seen.

History

A 47-year-old mother has been referred for a barium swallow study by her general practitioner (GP). She complains of increasing discomfort when eating and finds that food sometimes gets stuck in her throat. This is more often the case when eating meat or bread, and she finds that if she does not chew her food carefully, then each mouthful needs to be washed down with a glass of water. She has recently taken to eating soup for most meals, and does not find this too much of a problem. These symptoms have been getting very gradually worse over the past 5 months, and despite her change in diet she denies any significant weight loss.

There is no relevant past medical history, but her GP has recently prescribed iron tablets following a blood test for feelings of increasing lethargy. She attributes this to her heavy periods. She is a non-smoker and only drinks socially.

Examination

Her barium swallow study results are shown in Figure 66.1.

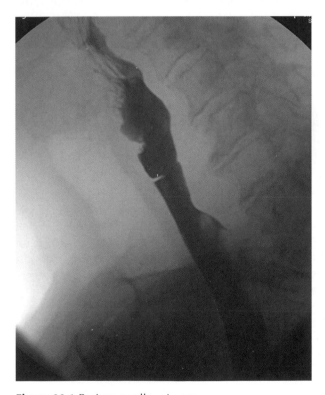

Figure 66.1 Barium swallow image.

Questions

- What does this view from the barium swallow show?
- What is the likely diagnosis?

ANSWER 66

For a barium swallow study, the patient is positioned between a fluoroscopy machine containing an X-ray tube and an image intensifier. This provides a real-time image that can be collimated to emphasize organs of the patient's neck and chest. The patient is asked to drink a contrast agent (e.g. barium) and hold it in the mouth. In coordination with the radiologist, asking the patient to swallow on command allows for good opacification of the oesophagus and direct real-time observation of the passage the contrast takes. Although many fluoroscopy studies are rarely used these days (e.g. barium enemas), swallow studies using barium or iodinated contrast medium are the 'workhorse' of foregut imaging. As a relatively non-invasive technique, it allows for accurate visualization of the oesophageal diameter and mucosa, and is often used to confirm the presence of persistent oesophageal leaks post-operatively.

This single lateral image is centred on the hypopharynx and upper oesophagus. Contrast passes freely from the mouth to the mid-oesophagus with no evidence of hold-up or obstruction. There is no evidence of aspiration. Within the proximal oesophagus at the level of C5, there is an anterior 'shelf-like' filling defect seen. This arises at right angles to the anterior oesophageal wall and appears to encroach into the oesophageal canal by approximately one-third. There is no transition delay of contrast, and no evidence of prestenotic dilatation or oesophageal diverticulosis. These features are in keeping with an oesophageal web.

Oesophageal webs are thin membranes of normal oesophageal squamous tissue that grow out from the anterior mucosal wall. Measuring approximately 1–2 mm in thickness, they can cause complete or incomplete circumferential narrowing of the oesophageal lumen and are most commonly seen in middle-aged white women. Symptoms are dependent on the degree of obstruction, with patients complaining of dysphagia for solids rather than liquids. Often found incidentally when patients present with feelings of globus or suffering food bolus impaction, symptoms can also include pain (odynophagia).

The aetiology of oesophageal webs is uncertain but can be both congenital, or more commonly, acquired. They are associated with chronic inflammatory conditions of the oesophagus including epidermolysis bullosa, pemphigus and bullous pemphigoid, and are also seen in coeliac and graft-versus-host disease. There is a strong association with Plummer–Vinson syndrome (PVS), in which patients experience concomitant glossitis, angular stomatitis and iron-deficiency anaemia. Image findings should always be correlated with a full blood count to exclude this.

Treatment of oesophageal webs is routinely performed with balloon dilatation, and is often a common byproduct of upper gastrointestinal endoscopy by bougienage. There is an increased association with oesophageal cancer, and recurrence of symptoms should be investigated early.

 KEY POINTS

- A barium swallow investigation is recommended for assessment of dysphagia.
- Oesophageal webs are thin membranes of normal oesophageal squamous tissue that grow out from the anterior mucosal wall.
- There is a strong correlation between oesophageal webs and other chronic inflammatory conditions.

History

A 24-year-old pregnant woman with hyperemesis presents to the accident and emergency department with chest pain and swelling around the neck after 3 days of worsening vomiting. She is dehydrated and breathless. She is in the 10th week of a confirmed intra-uterine twin pregnancy and has already attended the early pregnancy unit for treatment for vomiting. There has been no per vaginal (PV) bleeding or abnormal discharge. None of her close contacts have similar symptoms. Her medical history is otherwise unremarkable.

Examination

She appears dehydrated and mildly agitated but otherwise fit. Swelling over the lower neck and upper chest is noted that on palpation causes crepitus. She has mild tachycardia but no pyrexia. More crepitus is heard over the lungs. The heart sounds are normal. The abdomen is soft and mildly diffusely tender.

You arrange a chest radiograph (Figure 67.1) and blood tests.

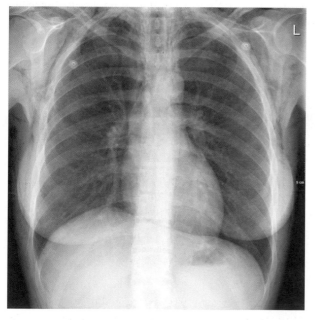

Figure 67.1 Posterior–anterior (PA) chest radiograph.

Questions

- What does the X-ray show?
- What imaging would you do next?
- What about the pregnancy?

The chest radiograph shows free gas within the upper mediastinum (i.e. a pneumomediastinum outlining the aorta and the trachea). There is also subcutaneous free gas (i.e. surgical emphysema), extending from the neck down over the upper thorax. No pneumothorax is seen. The lungs and heart appear normal.

Pneumomediastinum can be difficult to see on chest X-rays and is often missed if small. The characteristic appearances are streaky lucencies in the mediastinum, gas outlining structures such as vessels, pulmonary ligament and producing lucency between the hemidiaphragms. There may be associated pneumothoraces, pleural effusions, pneumopericardium or subcutaneous emphysema.

In terms of causes, it is useful to consider where the gas has come from. If it is intrathoracic, it could be from:

- oesophagus perforation secondary to foreign body, tumour or persistent vomiting (Boerhaave's syndrome);
- trachea or major bronchi – usually the result of blunt chest trauma, pneumothorax or tumours;
- lungs – due to alveolar rupture secondary to asthma in children, lung disease, ventilation or inhaled recreational drugs;
- pleural space – pneumothorax;
- iatrogenic causes – surgery, endoscopy or positive pressure ventilation;
- spontaneous – a cause is not found, typically in older patients.

If it is extrathoracic, it could be:

- head and neck – trauma, tumour, surgery;
- subdiaphragmatic – due to perforation of a viscus with gas tracking superiorly and through diaphragmatic openings.

Computed tomography (CT) is usually done if there is uncertainty about the radiograph and to see the extent of free gas (Figure 67.2).

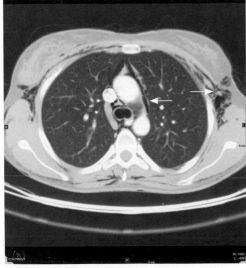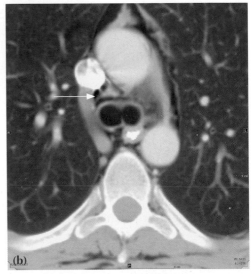

Figure 67.2 (a) Axial CT of the mediastinum showing mediastinal gas outlining the vessels and trachea and in the subcutaneous tissues (arrows); (b) enlarged view of the mediastinum.

If there is suspicion of oesophageal rupture, a water-soluble contrast swallow test should be done as there is a high risk for mediastinitis which has a poor prognosis (Figure 67.3).

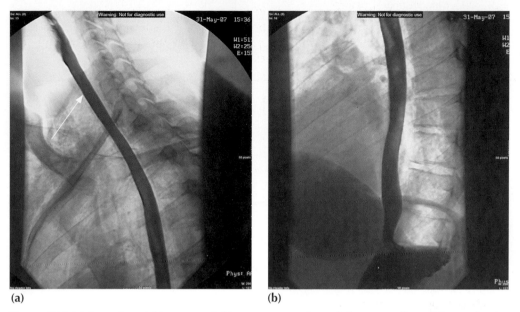

(a)   (b)

Figure 67.3 (a) Lateral and (b) water-soluble contrast swallow. Adjacent outline of the tracheal wall is seen due to interposed gas (arrow).

In Boerhaave's syndrome, where there is oesophageal rupture secondary to vomiting, the point of injury is typically in the left posterolateral wall a few centimetres above the gastro-oesophageal junction, and the largest amount of gas may be in the left side of the mediastinum. Neither of these signs is seen in Figure 67.3.

Rules governing licensing of radiology departments, which in the United Kingdom go under the name IRMER (Ionising Radiation (Medical Exposure) Regulations 2000), require a physician to justify the investigation, a technical member of the department to perform the investigation and a qualified person to review and report the outcome. In addition is the principle of the ALARP ('as low as reasonably possible') dose. In routine practice, people tend to think most about this when performing X-ray investigations on children or pregnant women. The reason is that certain types of tissue, typically rapidly growing or metabolically active tissue, is the most radiosensitive. It is worth remembering that some adult tissue remains more radiosensitive, in particular breast, gonads and thyroid.

The process of calculating radiation doses and including tissue sensitivities to produce an exposure that can be used in calculating risks is complicated and is often not required in such detail because the clinical risk associated with an uncertain diagnosis may be much higher (e.g. in pulmonary embolism). A few numbers are helpful to get a feel for comparative doses. Annual background is about 3 mSv, chest X-ray 0.02 mSv, abdomen 0.7 mSv, head CT 2 mSv, chest CT 8 mSv, abdominal/pelvis CT 10 mSv.

Justification for an investigation usually rests on the clinical risk of complications of a missed diagnosis, which are typically much larger than the long-term risk of X-ray exposure. In this case the surgical risk of mediastinitis and miscarriage justifies the exposure. The ALARP principle may have been used in deciding to do the contrast swallow first as a CT may not have been necessary if a leak had been demonstrated.

KEY POINTS

- Pneumomediastinum is easy to miss on a chest radiograph. Look for gas outlining the upper mediastinal structures.
- If oesophageal rupture is suspected, a contrast swallow should be performed as there is a high rate of mediastinitis and mortality.
- You need to be able to justify your investigations from a clinical and X-ray exposure point of view.

History

A 4-month-old boy is brought into the paediatric accident and emergency department by his parents with a head injury. The mother gives a history of the child falling from the changing table earlier in the day and explains the delay in coming to hospital on difficulties getting transport. The child otherwise has an unremarkable medical and neonatal history.

Examination

The child is listless but with normal observations. He responds to voice by eye opening but appears to move very little. He is probably a little under weight. There is a hard irregularity in the left parietal scalp but no laceration. The fontanelles are not bulging. There are no focal neurological signs. There appears to be some bruising over the left side of the chest and a swollen left finger.

You are suspicious about the extent of the injuries and about the behaviour of the father who appears to be keen to downplay the incident and leave. You discuss your concerns with the registrar who admits the patient, arranges skull and chest radiographs (Figure 68.1 and 68.2) and contacts the on-call social services to see if the child is on the at-risk register.

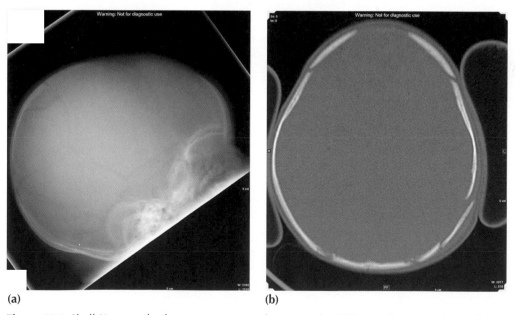

(a)   (b)

Figure 68.1 Skull X-ray and subsequent computed tomography (CT) scan (bone window) of the head.

While in the radiology department, the child becomes unresponsive and is intubated to maintain his airway.

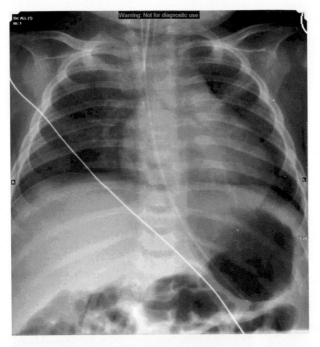

Figure 68.2 Chest radiograph post intubation and nasogastric (NG) tube insertion, windowed to optimize the bone appearance.

Questions

- What head injury does the child have?
- What else would you check for on the CT scan?
- Are further scans of the head indicated?
- Is there any sign of injury on the chest radiograph?
- What differential diagnoses should you consider?

The skull imaging shows a complex fracture of the left parietal bone extending from the vertex inferiorly with some displacement of the fractured fragments. Not shown but also apparent on the CT is a small subdural haemorrhage below the fracture. No signs of raised intracranial pressure such as bulging fontanelles and compressed cerebrospinal fluid (CSF) spaces are seen and the brain parenchyma and ventricles appear normal. The patient and images are reviewed by the neurosurgical centre.

On the chest radiograph, three posterior left rib fractures are seen overlying the heart shadow with associated callus formation. The chest otherwise appears normal.

The unsaid differential so far is non-accidental injury (NAI), however, it is important to consider the alternatives, if only to dismiss them, as the diagnosis of NAI has significant consequences. Other differentials include accidental trauma (but current injuries are not in proportion to the history), birth trauma (too long ago), osteogenesis imperfecta (no family history, no osteopenia seen) and rickets (requires imaging of long bone metaphyses).

Features that make NAI more likely are multiple fractures of varying ages, fractures inconsistent with age or history or in unusual positions, posterior (rather than lateral) rib fractures, metaphyseal corner fractures in children that have not started crawling/walking and skull fractures that are complex, multiple, cross-sutures or not in the parietal bone.

Once a diagnosis of NAI has been considered as possible, the child is admitted for treatment and retained on the ward. The findings and management are reviewed by the most senior paediatrician and social care services are immediately involved. In terms of further imaging, a skeletal survey is done to systematically document all and possible age of bony injuries. If the CT is abnormal or there are neurological symptoms or ongoing concern, brain magnetic resonance imaging (MRI) is done that may show subdural haematomas of varying ages or cortical contusions or shearing injuries from shaking injury. Delayed imaging may be helpful to show injuries acute at the time of presentation and not easily seen (Figure 68.3).

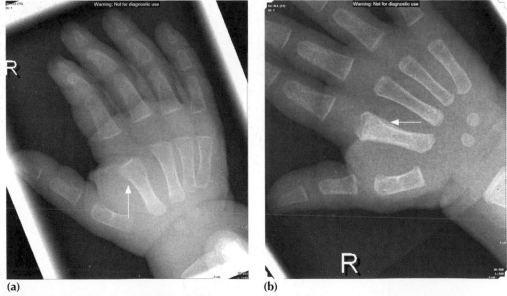

(a)   **(b)**

Figure 68.3 (a) Acute and (b) delayed images of the right hand showing a fracture of the second finger metacarpal (see arrows) with a step in image a) and sclerosis and periosteal reaction in b).

History

A 65-year-old woman presents to the accident and emergency department with vomiting.
She is known to have metastatic ovarian carcinoma with a large primary tumour that is
invading surrounding structures. There are lung and liver metastases. She has recently
completed a course of chemotherapy. She complains of a long history of variable bowel
habit and has not opened her bowels for the last 2 days.

Examination

She looks thin and in discomfort. There is mild dehydration, no fever and observations
are normal. She has a distended abdomen that is soft but generally tender. There are
hyperactive bowel sounds on auscultation. Her chest is clear and heart sounds are normal.

You arrange an abdominal radiograph (Figure 69.1), review the staging computed tomography (CT) scan of the pelvis from a few months previously that describes metastatic
masses and organize a water-soluble contrast enema (Figure 69.2).

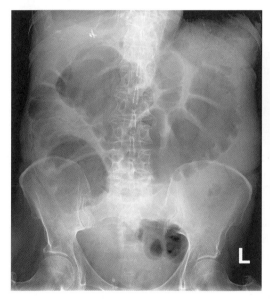

Figure 69.1 Abdominal radiograph.

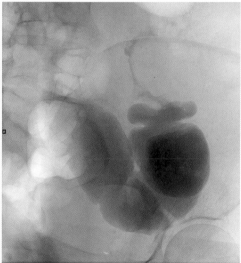

Figure 69.2 Water-soluble contrast enema.
Oblique projection of the sigmoid colon.

Questions

- What does the abdominal radiograph show?
- What does the enema show?
- Where does the problem lie?

The large bowel is investigated by introducing gas or contrast rectally, known as an enema. Barium enemas and CT colonograms require thorough bowel preparation and a bowel relaxant such as buscopan is given. In a barium enema, barium contrast is introduced into the bowel through a rectal tube and then mostly removed after coating the large bowel round to the caecum. Gas is then introduced to distend the bowel and radiographs are taken in several planes to view the entire bowel wall. In a CT colonogram, gas only is introduced to distend the bowel. Supine and prone scans are made with intravenous contrast.

A water-soluble contrast enema is typically used in acute situations where there is risk of perforation or likelihood of surgery, and does not require bowel preparation. Leakage of barium into the abdominal cavity runs a high risk of barium peritonitis, although in relatively healthy patients the risk is less than 1 in 3000.

The abdominal radiograph (Figure 69.1) shows gas within dilated bowel that demonstrates a haustral pattern (fold involving only part of the bowel wall) characteristic of large bowel. The position is typical of the caecum and transverse colon with only a small amount of gas in the descending and sigmoid colon. No gas is seen in the small bowel, suggesting the terminal ileal valve is patent. The dilated bowel pattern suggests there is an obstruction at the splenic flexure level.

In the water-soluble contrast enema (Figure 69.2), contrast was seen to flow through the rectum, and into the sigmoid colon. Contrast passed no further than the mid-sigmoid colon where a stricture was seen. The imaging suggests two strictures postioned in the descending and mid-sigmoid colon.

The history and staging CT indicate that there is metastatic ovarian disease. Ovarian carcinoma is the second most common gynaecological malignancy and fifth leading cause of cancer deaths in women. Risk factors include nulliparity, early menarche, late menopause and positive family history of ovarian, breast and early colorectal cancer. It is often discovered late as abdominal symptoms of pain and distension, bowel habit change, urinary frequency are often intermittent, non-specific and dismissed as common abdominal twinges. The tumour spreads by direct extension, intraperitoneal implantation (often with ascites to produce omental deposits or 'omental cake') and lymphatic and haematogenous spread, commonly to liver and lung. In this patient, there is bowel obstruction remote from the tumour that invades the sigmoid colon and this may reflect intraperitoneal implantation.

There are two aspects to this patient's treatment. One is to relieve the immediate problem of obstruction and the other is treating the underlying disease. With widespread metastases the underlying disease is treated with chemo- and radiotherapy. The obstruction is treated by palliative surgery to create a colostomy or stent insertion.

Increasingly stents are being used for palliative treatment of strictures using either fluoroscopy (movable X-ray camera) or endoscopy to pass a wire through the stricture and then fluoroscopy to insert the stent.

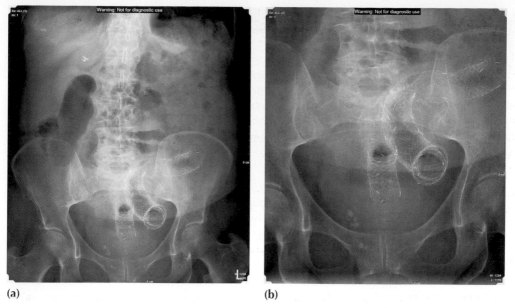

(a) (b)

Figure 69.3 Abdominal radiograph showing stents in the rectosigmoid and descending colon.

🔑 **KEY POINTS**

- Bowel obstruction can be diagnosed if there is a transition point, where the bowel size changes due to an intrinsic or extrinsic cause.
- Water-soluble contrast enemas are used in acute situations where the risk of perforation or imminent surgery is high.
- Stents can be used to treat strictures, particularly in palliative care.

History

A 48-year-old woman attends her general practitioner (GP) having noticed a lump in her left breast while showering. The lump was non-tender and there had been no associated discharge. She took no medication. She had never taken the oral contraceptive pill and although recently post-menopausal, she had never taken hormone replacement therapy. There was no family history of breast cancer. She was otherwise fit and well with no previous medical or surgical history.

Examination

On examination there is a firm mass laterally and superiorly (in the upper outer quadrant). There are no overlying skin changes, but the mass felt firm and moves when tensing the pectoral muscles and asking the patient to raise her hands above her head. There is also evidence of palpable left axillary lymph nodes. She is referred to the local breast service symptomatic clinic. On arrival she has a standard set of mammograms taken (Figures 70.1 and 70.2).

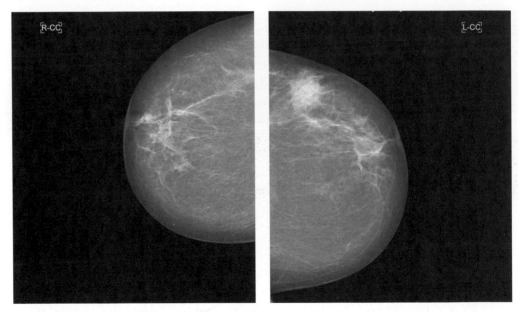

Figure 70.1 Standard cranial–caudal mammograms.

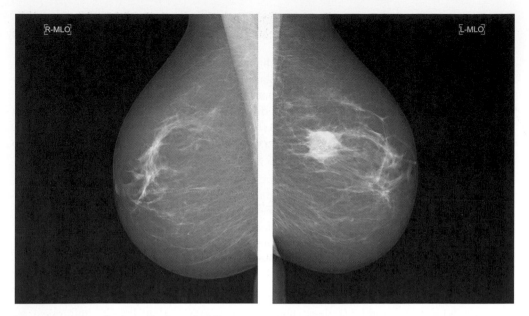

Figure 70.2 Standard medio-lateral-oblique mammograms.

Questions

- What do you notice on the mammograms?
- Which age group of women attend breast screening?
- What does the ultrasound in Figure 70.3 demonstrate?

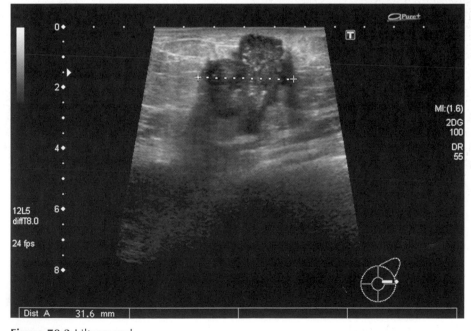

Figure 70.3 Ultrasound.

The cranial–caudal (CC) and medio-lateral-oblique (MLO) views shown in Figures 70.1b and 70.2b, respectively, demonstrate a large irregular, spiculate tumour containing microcalcifications. The lesion is located lateral (see CC view) and slightly superior (see MLO view) to the nipple in approximately the 2 o'clock position in the left breast. This is the typical appearance of a malignant breast carcinoma. For comparison the corresponding mammograms of the normal right breast are included in Figures 70.1a and 70.2a. The mass is causing parenchymal distortion and extends posteriorly, hence explaining some fixation seen on clinical examination.

Mammography can be performed both in the context of screening (in the asymptomatic woman) or diagnosis in the symptomatic patient. Until recently, women in the United Kingdom were invited to attend breast screening from age 50 with a 3-year cycle and continued to age 70. This has now been extended from 47 to 73 with self or GP referral for older women. In younger, typically pre-menopausal women the breast tissue is denser, making mammography less sensitive as a screening tool.

If an abnormality is found on screening it is graded, which determines the type of follow-up. Suspicious lesions are referred to a breast clinic. The standard breast mammogram views are bilateral CC and MLO views, which are obtained with the breast compressed, as seen in Figures 70.1 and 70.2.

Mammography is a form of low-dose radiograph used to create detailed images of the breast and can demonstrate microcalcifications smaller than 100 µm. It may reveal a lesion before it is palpable by examination, hence its use in screening. Mammographic features suggestive of malignancy include microcalcifications, soft tissue mass, asymmetry or architectural distortion, all of which are demonstrated in Figure 70.1b.

In the breast clinic the patient undergoes a triple assessment of clinical review, mammography and ultrasound. The ultrasound shown in Figure 70.3 confirms a 3.1 cm mass with ill-defined margins, casting an acoustic shadow. Ultrasound is a useful adjunct to mammography and has the benefit of not using ionizing radiation. Ultrasound can help to determine if a breast lesion is likely to be benign (e.g. a cyst or fibroadenoma) or malignant. Malignant lesions are characteristically poorly defined with irregular margins and posterior acoustic shadowing, as seen in Figure 70.3. Ultrasound is also used to guide biopsy and therapeutic procedures. In this patient's case, the lesion was an invasive ductal carcinoma.

In certain settings magnetic resonance (MR) imaging of the breast may be indicated. This is used for:

- further characterization of an indeterminate lesion (despite full assessment with examination, mammography and ultrasound);
- detection of occult breast carcinoma in a patient with carcinoma in an axillary lymph node;
- multifocal or bilateral tumours;
- invasive lobular carcinoma, which has a high incidence of multifocality;
- evaluation of suspected, extensive, high-grade intraductal carcinoma;
- detection of recurrent breast cancer.

 KEY POINTS

- Breast clinic assessment typically consists of the triple assessment of clinical review, mammography and ultrasound.
- Mammography can be used both in screening and in symptomatic presentations such as a breast lump or discharge.
- Ultrasound can be used to characterize breast lesions and guide biopsy.

History

A 57-year-old man was admitted overnight complaining of haematuria and lethargy. His symptoms have been intermittent over the last month, with occasional macroscopic blood seen when passing urine. He complains of an increase in frequency and nocturia but no dysuria. There is no history to suggest any stigmata of infection.

He has no relevant past medical history and lives at home with his wife and two children. As an ex-smoker he has a tobacco history of 20 pack-years with only occasional alcohol usage.

Examination

Examination reveals that he is afebrile and in no obvious discomfort. Cardiovascular and respiratory examinations are normal, but on abdominal examination there is fullness at both renal angles and mild discomfort on deep palpation.

Blood results reveal a creatinine of 515 µmol/L with normal urea and potassium. A routine blood result from 3 months previously recorded his creatinine as 72 µmol/L. His inflammatory markers are not elevated and a blood gas does not demonstrate any acidosis. Ultrasound images were taken (Figures 71.1 and 71.2).

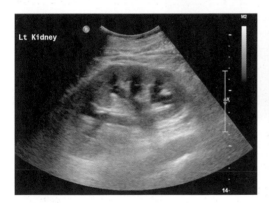

Figure 71.1 Ultrasound of left kidney.

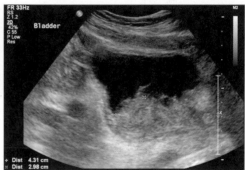

Figure 71.2 Ultrasound of bladder.

Questions

- What does the ultrasound show?
- What options are available to resolve the situation?

These are two static ultrasound images of the left kidney and the bladder. The left kidney image is acquired in a longitudinal orientation and demonstrates normal echogenicity and shape with preserved corticomedullary differentiation and cortical thickness. There are serpiginous areas of anechoic echogenicity associated with the renal medulla with cortical extension in keeping with moderate pelivocalyceal dilatation (Figure 71.3). Although not accurately demonstrated on this image, there is the suggestion of proximal ureteric dilatation distal to the pelvico-ureteric junction (PUJ). Imaging of the right kidney revealed identical appearances.

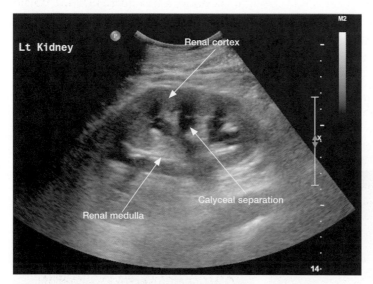

Figure 71.3 Annotated ultrasound of left kidney.

The second image (Figure 71.2) is acquired in a transverse orientation within the pelvis and demonstrates an adequately distended bladder with an area of irregular echogenicity seen posteriorly at the expected level of the bladder trigone. This mass lesion measures approximately 4.3 × 2.9 cm contiguous with the bladder wall. The vesico-ureteric junction (VUJ) and distal ureters are not demonstrated on this image. The features are likely to represent a transitional cell carcinoma (TCC) of the bladder with obstruction of both the left and right kidneys. A staging computed tomography (CT) examination of the chest, abdomen and bladder is recommended to characterize this further, with referral to a urologist for continued management.

The CT scan confirmed a surgically resectable TCC with bilateral renal obstruction and no evidence of local or distant spread. The patient ultimately requires a definitive surgical procedure to remove the cancer, but at present, the ureteric obstruction and deterioration in renal function makes the patient biochemically unstable. Surgery carries significant risk, and in a non-life threatening situation, the patient should be physically and bio-chemically optimized to encourage a safe transition through the operation, reduce the risk of intra-operative mortality and improve post-operative recovery. This patient is currently a poor candidate for general anaesthesia, and as a bridge to surgery there are two options available:

- **Cystoscopy and retrograde ureteric stent insertion:** Trained urologists can pass a camera through the patient's urethra and visualize the bladder TCC directly. Not only does this allow for biopsy and tissue confirmation of the TCC, but if the VUJ is adequately visualized, a guidewire can be passed into the ureter and a 'double-J' stent inserted to relieve the VUJ obstruction. Cystoscopy can be performed under conscious sedation but general anaesthesia is preferred. In this situation, it was felt that the tumour mass would make VUJ cannulation very difficult, making this option inappropriate.
- **Nephrostomy and antegrade ureteric stent insertion:** This minimally invasive procedure is performed by a trained interventional radiologist and can be performed under local anaesthesia only, although light sedation is sometimes required. The patient lies on a fluoroscopy table in the prone position, and a micropuncture needle is passed percutaneously under direct ultrasound imaging into a dilated lower pole calyx. Ideally this should transgress Brodel's bloodless line, an avascular area between the anterior and posterior renal segments to reduce the risk of renal haemorrhage. Instilling contrast into the collecting system under fluoroscopy can confirm satisfactory positioning (Figure 71.4).

Adopting the Seldinger technique, a guidewire can then be manipulated into the proximal ureter over which a sheath is passed to stabilize the position. A hydrophilic wire and catheter combination is then used to transgress the VUJ and obstructing lesion for safe passage of a stiff guidewire from the renal pelvis into the bladder. This allows careful manipulation of an appropriately sized renal stent to be passed over the wire so that one end lies within the bladder, and the other lies more proximally within the renal pelvis. This acts as a conduit through which urine can drain for renal decompression (Figure 71.5).

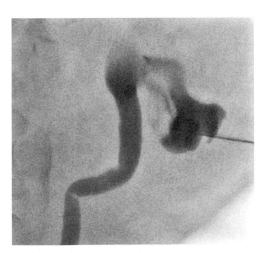

Figure 71.4 Contrast fluoroscopy image confirming position of lower pole colyx.

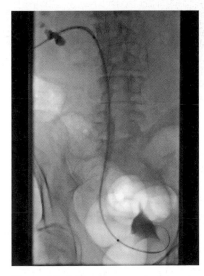

Figure 71.5 Fluoroscopy study positioning ureteric stent.

Stent positioning requires a high level of accuracy and it may also become obstructed both by tumour overgrowth and stent migration. As a precautionary measure, an additional pigtail catheter is often left within the renal pelvis, running along the line of the original percutaneous puncture to act as a urinary diversion both for initial decompression and in case of stent failure. This is termed a covering nephrostomy and remains in position for the short term (Figure 71.6).

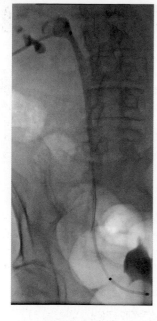

Figure 71.6 Fluoroscopy image confirming ureteric stent placement with covering nephrostomy.

Renal decompression will allow time for the renal function to return to normal and means that the operation can be performed in a less urgent and more controlled environment. Holistically, it also allows for the patient to make appropriate decisions about their own management. The nephrostomy and stent can be removed intra-operatively, leaving only a small cutaneous scar.

 KEY POINTS

- Nephrostomy allows for biochemical and physical optimization before surgery.
- Nephrostomy insertion is ideally along Brodel's bloodless line.
- Ultrasound guidance and a Seldinger technique are employed for nephrostomy insertion.

History

A 21-year-old woman is brought to the accident and emergency department with head and neck trauma after falling from a horse. She is immobilized on a board with a hard neck collar and complains of diffuse neck pain and mild intermittent tingling in the arms and legs. There is no history of loss of consciousness, no evidence of head injury (she had a riding helmet on) and no complaint of injury elsewhere. There is no significant past medical history although the patient has had intermittent neck pain in the past that has not been investigated.

Examination

Routine observations are stable and she is maintaining her airway, breathing and circulation. You perform a primary survey which reveals diffuse tenderness in the mid cervical spine. There is abnormal sensation and hyperreflexia in lower and upper limbs. The chest, abdomen and pelvis are normal. No limb fractures or dislocations are suspected. You arrange trauma series radiographs of the neck (Figure 72.1).

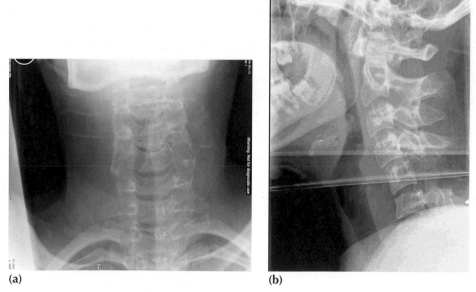

(a)   (b)

Figure 72.1 (a) Anterior–posterior (AP) and (b) lateral cervical spine views from the trauma series (normal AP peg view not shown). There is overlying artefact as the images are obtained with immobilization blocks.

Questions

- Which lines do you review on cervical spine radiographs?
- Is there an abnormality on the radiograph?
- Do you have a differential diagnosis?
- What would you do next?

A trauma series of cervical spine radiographs includes a peg view of the dens through the open mouth and various other views to ensure the C7/T1 junction is seen. If clear views are not obtained or an acute abnormality is noted then a computed tomography (CT) scan is the next step.

When assessing cervical spine radiographs, there are a number of lines that should be viewed to help pick up abnormalities. On the lateral projection, the anterior and posterior vertebral edges describe lines. The line through the junction of the lamina and the anterior edge of the spinous processes (spinolaminar line) and the curve through the posterior tips of the spinous processes should be reviewed. These lines should all be smooth and continuous with no steps, although the natural curvature of the neck may be altered due to pain or immobilization. Any small fragments of bone should be considered for fractures although may be ossification centres in younger patients or degenerative changes in older patients. On the AP view look at the lines through and spacing between the spinous processes and the pedicles.

The radiographs show a gap in the spinolaminar line at C5 with absence of a normal spinous process and an expanded appearance of both pedicles and lamina, best seen on the AP projection. The anterior and posterior vertebral lines appear normal. No fracture is identified, however, the appearance suggests a chronic expansile bone lesion involving the pedicles and spinous process of C5 that may be narrowing the spinal canal. No significant soft tissue swelling or periosteal reaction is seen to suggest an aggressive process.

In the absence of a fracture, the patient's acute symptoms are likely to be due to cord trauma secondary to spinal stenosis (narrowing) that may be due to the underlying bone lesion or a new haematoma. Spinal stenosis can be congenital or acquired and most often affects the cervical or lumbar spine. Degenerative change or metastatic bone lesions are common causes in patients over 50. Congenital or acquired primary bone lesions as well as trauma are more common in younger patients.

A CT is required to characterize the bone changes and ensure there is no traumatic injury (Figure 72.2).

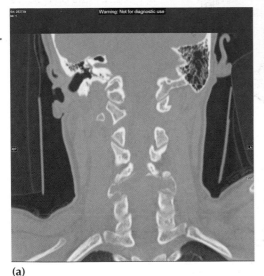 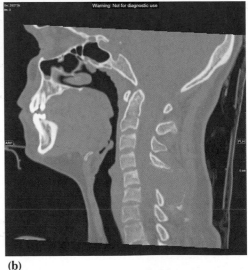

(a)   **(b)**

Figure 72.2 (a) Coronal and (b) sagittal images of the patient's cervical spine showing the expansile lesion in the posterior elements of the C5 vertebra. No fracture is seen.

Given the patient's neurology, an emergency magnetic resonance (MR) scan is required to examine the spinal cord, nerve roots and soft tissue associated with the bone lesion (Figure 72.3).

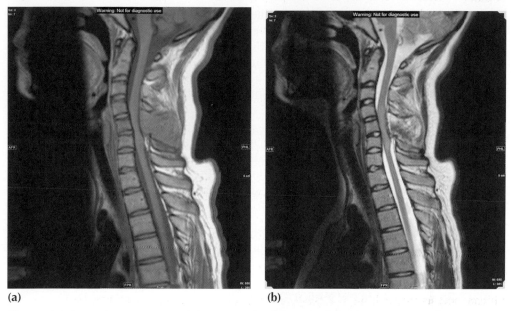

(a)   (b)

Figure 72.3 Sagittal MR (a) T1- and (b) T2-weighted images of the patient's cervical spine.

The MR shows an expansile lesion of the C5 spinous process with associated narrowing of the spinal canal and increased T2 signal (altered water content) within the spinal canal at this point. The high signal is most likely to be inflammatory due to trauma and cord swelling rather than a tumour or haemorrhage.

Given the patient's age, possible differential diagnoses for expansile lesions in the cervical spine include benign tumours from the bone such as an aneurysmal bone cyst, as in this case, or from the spinal cord or nerve roots such as a neurofibroma. Malignant bone tumours are less likely given the age and history but could include lymphoma. Osteomyelitis should also be ruled out although unlikely in this case.

The patient requires urgent referral to a neurosurgical/spinal orthopaedic centre for possible removal of the lesion to decompress the cord. Steroids may help to reduce cord swelling.

KEY POINTS

- Acute or symptomatic spinal stenosis is an emergency and one of the few situations requiring an emergency MR to view the cord.
- Degenerative changes and disc prolapse are the most common causes of spinal stenosis, but the differential includes tumours and haematomas.

History

This 25-year-old man presents to you in the accident and emergency department with lower back pain that is so bad he is unable to walk. He gives a history of gradually worsening back pain over the last few months. He also complains of night sweats and bowel disturbance. He does not give a history of other medical problems and says that he is not working currently. He smokes 15 cigarettes a day and drinks at least 30 units a week. He takes cannabis regularly but denies use of intravenous drugs.

Examination

On examination he is thin and appears to neglect his appearance. His blood pressure, pulse and temperature are a little elevated. His chest and heart sounds are normal. The abdomen is soft. There is evidence of injection sites in the forearms and antecubital fossae. He is extremely tender over the lower spine. Neurologically, he has reduced power (4/5) on leg raising bilaterally.

You arrange investigations including a chest and lumbar spine radiograph (Figure 73.1) and, on the basis of that, a magnetic resonance (MR) scan of the spine is arranged (Figure 73.2).

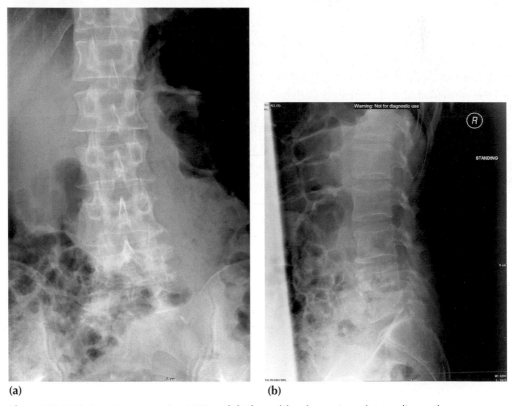

(a)   **(b)**

Figure 73.1 (a) Anterior–posterior (AP) and (b) lateral lumbar spine plain radiographs.

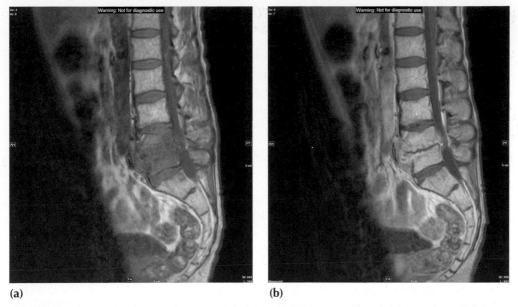

(a)　　　　　　　　　　　　　　　　　　　**(b)**

Figure 73.2 T1-weighted sagittal MR image of the lumbar spine, pre (a) and post (b) gadolinium contrast.

Just to give a brief summary of MR, hydrogen is a ubiquitous atom present in water and most biological molecules. In a magnetic field, the magnetic moment of the hydrogen nucleus becomes polarized and can be switched between aligned parallel and antiparallel with the magnetic field by radiofrequency pulses. Add in a magnetic field gradient to change the frequency at which the protons resonate according to position and you have the beginnings of spatial resolution and an MR image.

The protons relax from an ordered polarized state once the radiofrequency pulse has stopped. The relaxation of polarization is measured with the T1 rate constant, and the rate at which they become disorganized by T2. T1 and T2 are used as contrast parameters.

Fat and proteinaceous fluid have high T1 and T2 signals. Water has low T1and high T2 signal. Soft tissues are somewhere inbetween. Abnormalities often have high T2 signal. T1 images tend to be used for anatomy, comparison with T2 images or used with gadolinium contrast (high T1 signal).

Questions
- What do the figures demonstrate?
- Why was an MR scan ordered?
- What is the differential diagnosis.
- What would you do next and how?
- What is the appropriate treatment?

The plain radiograph (Figure 73.1) shows loss of disc and vertebral height at L4 and L5.

In many ways the MR images (Figure 73.2) complement the plain radiograph. Although the bone cortex appears dark, the marrow is bright due to fat. Loss of normal fat signal in L4 and 5 vertebral bodies results from inflammation and increased water signal. Contrast enhancement also reflects the pathological processes centred on the disc and affecting the bone. MR is also excellent for looking at soft tissues, particularly in this case the anterior paravertebral soft tissue mass as well as soft tissue impinging into the spinal canal and on to the nerve roots and the spinal cord itself.

With this patient's history there is a risk of immune suppression and a high risk of infection and the most likely diagnosis is infective discitis. Despite his denial, the injection marks without any other explanation makes it likely that he uses intravenous drugs. The differential diagnosis of malignancy is quite unlikely as this tends to affect primarily the vertebra. Osteomyelitis is also a differential if there is not disc involvement, however, in this case it is coexistent with the discitis.

Infection in the spine is typically the result of either bloodborne spread or through an invasive procedure. Infections can be either pyogenic or non-pyogenic. Pyogenic discitis most commonly involves *Staphylococcus aureus* or gram-negative bacilli in intravenous drug users or immunocompromised patients. Non-pyogenic discitis may be caused by tuberculosis (TB).

In children, where there is still vascularization of the disc, the infection arises in the disc. In adults, the infection arises in the vertebral endplate and then crosses the disc to the next endplate. Typical changes seen on imaging include loss of disc height and increasing loss of vertebral endplates with destruction and collapse. There may be formation of adjacent soft tissue masses or collections that may, particularly in TB, spread beneath the longitudinal ligaments to involve multiple levels.

Diagnosis typically requires identification of the organism. In some cases this may be secondary to infection or a collection elsewhere and identified on blood or other sample culture. Otherwise a biopsy is required to obtain some infected tissue. This is typically done using image-guided needle biopsy to negotiate the nerve roots and position the needle tip in the optimum position (Figure 73.3). This patient's biopsy yielded TB.

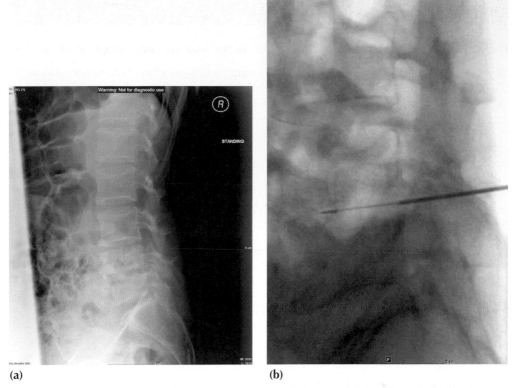

(a)

(b)

Figure 73.3 Fluoroscopic (movable X-ray camera)-guided biopsy of the affected disc showing the needle position.

History

An 11-year-old boy is playing at an adventure park when he falls on the climbing frame, catching his left thumb as he lands. There is immediate pain and swelling and he is unable to move his thumb. His mother takes him to the local accident and emergency department for evaluation.

Examination

He is distressed. His thumb is swollen with bony tenderness maximal in the region of the thumb proximal pharynx and metacarpal. There is virtually no range of movement at the thumb metacarpophalangeal joint or the interphalangeal joint. Capillary refill is normal (less than 2 seconds) and sensation is intact distally. A request is filled out for trauma views of the thumb to exclude a suspected fracture. The radiographs are seen in Figure 74.1.

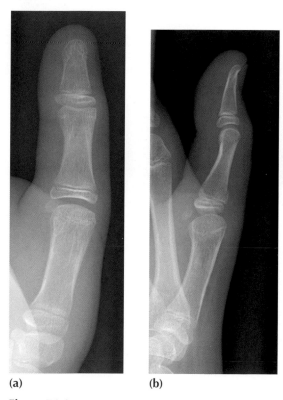

(a) (b)

Figure 74.1

Question

- What do the trauma views of the thumb demonstrate?

On the first radiograph (Figure 74.1a) it is difficult to appreciate a bony injury, but the second trauma view (Figure 74.1b) clearly demonstrates a fracture line passing through the base of the thumb proximal phalynx metaphysis into the epiphyseal plate. The fracture line does not, however, pass through into the epiphysis. This is the classical appearance of a Salter–Harris type II fracture.

Salter–Harris fractures are fractures through a growth plate and, as a result, unique to paediatric patients. They are common injuries found in children, occurring in approximately 15 per cent of long bone fractures. These fractures are classified according to the involvement of the physis, metaphysis and epiphysis. This categorization of the injuries is important because it not only affects patient treatment but may also alert the clinician to potential longer term complications.

There are nine types of Salter–Harris fracture in total, although types I–V are the most commonly referred to and were those described originally (the rarer types VI–IX have been added subsequently). The radiographic findings vary according to the type of Salter–Harris fracture.

The most common type of Salter–Harris fracture, is the type II fracture (see arrow Figure 74.2). This occurs through the physis and metaphysis, and the epiphysis is not involved in the injury (no fracture is observed in the epiphysis).

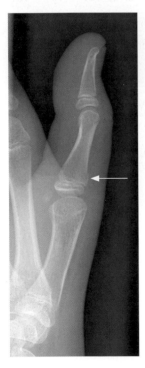

Figure 74.2

Salter–Harris type II fractures tend to occur after age 10. The mechanism involves shearing or avulsion with angular force. There is cartilage failure on the tension side. Metapetaphyseal failure occurs on the compression side. There is a division between epiphysis and metaphysis except for a flake of metaphyseal bone, which is carried with the epiphysis. The metaphyseal fragment is sometimes called the Thurston–Holland fragment. These fractures may cause minimal shortening, however healing is usually rapid and Salter–Harris type II injuries rarely result in functional limitations.

With type I Salter–Harris fractures, initial radiographs may suggest separation of the physis although this separation may not be apparent and soft tissue swelling typically overlying the physis may provide the only clue. Follow-up radiographs within 2 weeks after injury help establish the diagnosis. Adjacent sclerosis and/or periosteal reaction along the epiphyseal plate supports the diagnosis of a Salter–Harris type I fracture. The growing physis is not usually injured in type I fractures, however, and growth disturbance is uncommon.

The type III fracture passes through the physis and extends to split the epiphysis. The fracture crosses the physis and extends into the articular surface of the bone. Type IV injuries pass through the epiphysis, physis and metaphysis. As with type III fractures, the type IV pattern is an intra-articular injury and therefore can result in chronic disability. Type V fractures are compression/crush injuries of the epiphyseal plate, without associated epiphyseal or metaphyseal fracture. The initial plain radiographs in type V fracture may not show a fracture line (similar to type I fractures). Soft-tissue swelling at the physis, however, is usually present. The clinical history is central to the diagnosis of type V fractures and a typical history is that of an axial load injury. Type V injuries have a poor functional prognosis.

 KEY POINTS

- Salter–Harris fractures are fractures through a growth plate.
- Imaging findings vary according to the type of Salter–Harris fracture.
- The most common type of Salter-Harris fracture is the type II fracture which occurs through the physis and metaphysis (the epiphysis is not involved in the injury).
- The diagnosis of type V may be particularly difficult, however is important as these injuries have a poor functional prognosis.
- Two views are required in the evaluation of all cases of traumatic injury.

History

A 60-year-old man presents to his general practitioner (GP). Over the course of the last month he has noted bright red blood in his urine. He had hoped that it would simply go away but instead he has now developed loin discomfort, particularly on the right. He has not felt feverish or lost any weight. He is an ex-smoker and takes antihypertensive medication, but otherwise he has been well.

Examination

He was afebrile and his observations were all within normal limits. Upon palpation the abdomen was soft and no mass was felt. There was tenderness in the right renal angle but no direct pain on palpation. His white cell count was slightly elevated at 13×10^9/L and his C-reactive protein (CRP) is 20 mg/L. He also demonstrates a mild normocytic anaemia with a haemoglobin of 10.4 g/dL. Urine dipstick reveals frank blood. He is referred for an ultrasound scan which is reported as 'bilateral hydronephrosis, although the bladder was suboptimally distended therefore could not be completely evaluated.' One longitudinal image of the right kidney is seen in Figure 75.1. On the basis of the ultrasound scan, further imaging with computed tomography (CT) was arranged with the local radiology department. A coronal reconstructed image is seen in Figure 75.2.

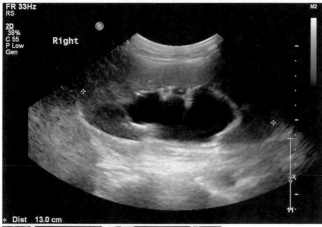

Figure 75.1 Ultrasound image.

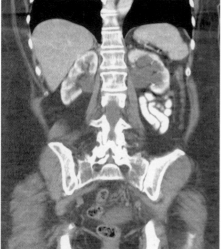

Question

- What do the ultrasound image in Figure 75.1 and the CT image in Figure 75.2 demonstrate?

Figure 75.2 CT scan.

Figure 75.1 demonstrates dilatation of the right renal pelvicalyceal system consistent with hydronephrosis. Compare this appearance with that of a normal unobstructed kidney in Figure 75.3.

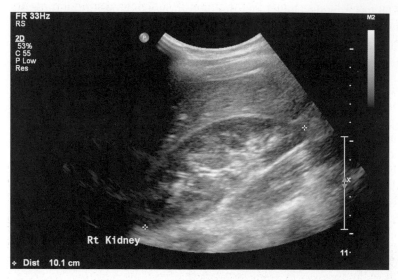

Figure 75.3 Ultrasound of normal kidney.

Figure 75.2 shows a coronal contrast-enhanced CT image demonstrating dilatation of the renal collecting system bilaterally.

This patient has bilateral hydronephrosis (seen on ultrasound and CT) in combination with frank haematuria. A cystoscopy was then arranged which confirmed the presence of a bladder lesion obstructing both ureteric orifices.

Hydronephrosis is distension and dilatation of the renal pelvis calyces, usually caused by the obstruction of the free flow of urine from the kidney(s), and may lead to progressive atrophy of the kidney(s). This case demonstrates only one cause of hydronephrosis.

A multitude of causes exist for hydronephrosis and hydroureter, ranging from benign processes, such as the physiologic hydroureteronephrosis of pregnancy, to potential life-threatening situations, such as infected hydronephrosis or pyonephrosis. Classification can be made according to the level within the urinary tract (interruption can occur anywhere along the urinary tract from the kidneys to the urethral meatus) and whether the aetiology is intrinsic, extrinsic or functional. Causes at ureteric level can be intrinsic (for example, ureteropelvic junction stricture, blood clot, retrocaval ureter), functional (for example, gram-negative infection or neurogenic bladder) or extrinsic (for example, retroperitoneal or pelvic malignancy or pregnancy). At the level of the bladder intrinsic causes include carcinoma (as in this case), calculi, cystocele or diverticula; functional causes include vesico-ureteric reflux; and extrinsic causes again include malignancy and pelvic lipomatosis. Urethral causes may also be intrinsic, such as strictures or valves, or extrinsic, such as prostatic pathology.

Although patients usually present with signs or symptoms, hydronephrosis can be an incidental finding encountered during the evaluation of an unrelated process.

Hydronephrosis that occurs acutely with sudden onset (for example, due to a renal calculus) can cause intense pain in the flank area, while a chronic occurrence that develops gradually will present with no pain or attacks of a dull discomfort. Nausea and vomiting may also occur. An obstruction that occurs at the urethra or bladder outlet can cause pain and pressure resulting from distension of the bladder. Blocking the flow of urine will commonly result in urinary tract infections which can lead to the development of additional stones, fever, and blood or pus in the urine. If complete obstruction occurs, kidney failure may follow.

If unrecognized or left untreated, hydronephrosis/hydroureter secondary to obstruction can lead to hypertension, loss of renal function, and sepsis. Consequently, patients found to have hydronephrosis or hydroureter should undergo a thorough evaluation. The specific treatment of a patient with hydronephrosis depends on the aetiology of the process, with any signs of infection within the obstructed system warranting urgent intervention (as infection of an obstructed system may progress rapidly to sepsis).

 KEY POINTS

- The appearances of hydronephrosis on ultrasound or CT are of a dilated renal pelvis and calyceal system.
- A multitude of causes exist, with classification made according to the level within the urinary tract and whether the aetiology is intrinsic, extrinsic or functional.
- Treatment of hydronephrosis focuses upon the removal of the obstruction and/or drainage of the urine that has accumulated behind the obstruction.
- Any sign of infection within an obstructed system should prompt urgent intervention.

History

A 63-year-old man is lifting boxes at home when he experiences the sudden onset of lower back pain. The pain is so severe that he is unable to move and consequently calls an ambulance. Upon admission to accident and emergency he describes the pain as sharp and radiating down his legs, more severe on the left.

Examination

On examination there are reduced ankle reflexes and weakness of plantar flexion at the ankle on both sides. He is unable to straight leg raise on the left. He is admitted under the orthopaedic team for management of the pain and a magnetic resonance imaging (MRI) scan is performed (Figures 76.1 and 76.2).

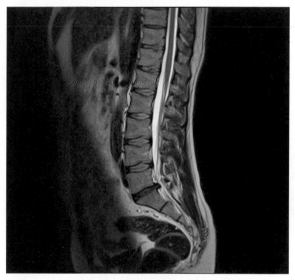

Figure 76.1 Sagittal T2-weighted MR image of the lumbar-sacral spine.

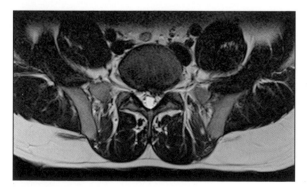

Figure 76.2 Axial T2-weighted MR image.

Questions

- What do the MRI images show?
- What is the reason for these appearances?

Figure 76.1 is a sagittal T2-weighted MR image of the lumbar-sacral spine, which demonstrates a disc prolapse at the level of L5/S1. Figure 76.2 is an axial T2-weighted MR image through the level of the disc herniation, which demonstrates the disc effacing the left L5 nerve root as it exits the spinal canal.

A spinal disc herniation is a medical condition affecting the spine, in which a tear in the outer, fibrous ring (annulus fibrosus) of an intervertebral disc allows the soft, central portion (nucleus pulposus) to bulge out. Tears are frequently posterolateral owing to the presence of the posterior longitudinal ligament in the spinal canal. Nuclear material that is displaced into the spinal canal is associated with an inflammatory response, and the tear in the disc ring can result in the release of inflammatory chemical mediators which may directly cause pain, even in the absence of nerve root compression. This is the rationale for using anti-inflammatory medication for pain associated with disc herniation, protrusion, bulge or disc tear.

A weakened annulus is a necessary condition for herniation to occur. Many cases involve trivial trauma, sometimes in the presence of repetitive stress. Traumatic injury to lumbar discs commonly occurs when lifting while bent at the waist, rather than lifting with the legs while the back is straight.

Lumbar disc herniations occur most often between the fourth and fifth lumbar vertebral bodies or between L5 and the S1 (as in this example). Symptoms can affect the lower back, buttocks, thigh, anal or genital region (via the perineal nerve) and may radiate into the foot. The sciatic nerve is the most commonly affected nerve, causing symptoms of sciatica. The femoral nerve may also be affected.

Plain radiographs do not demonstrate disc herniation but are useful in the diagnosis of other conditions, particularly fracture, bone metastases or infection, and should be the primary imaging modality when trauma, malignancy or infection are suspected.

MR imaging is the modality of choice for delineating herniated nucleus pulposus and its relationship with adjacent soft tissues. On MRI, disc prolapses appear as focal, asymmetric protrusions of disc material beyond the confines of the annulus. Herniation of the nucleus pulposus are usually hypo-intense, however, because disc herniations are often associated with a radial annular tear, high signal intensity in the posterior annulus is often seen on sagittal T2-weighted images.

On sagittal MR images the relationship of herniation of the nucleus pulposus and degenerated facets to exiting nerve roots within the neural foramina is well delineated. In addition, free fragments of the disc are easily detected on MRI.

In cases of disc bulging, early MR findings include loss of the normal posterior disc concavity. Moderate bulges appear as non-focal protrusions of disc material beyond the borders of the vertebrae. Bulges are typically broad based, circumferential and symmetric.

A radial tear of the annulus fibrosus is considered a sign of early disc degeneration. It is accompanied by other signs of disc degeneration, such as a bulging annulus, loss of disc height, herniation of the nucleus pulposus and changes in the adjacent endplates.

 KEY POINTS

- Herniation of the nucleus pulposus through an annular defect causes focal protrusion of the disc material beyond the margins of the adjacent vertebral endplate.
- MR imaging is the modality of choice for demonstrating the relationship of the herniated nucleus pulposus and degenerated facets to exiting nerve roots within the neural foramina.

History

A 30-year-old woman is admitted to hospital with a fever and a cough. She has a history of repeated chest infections for several years, two of which have required hospital admission. She has been coughing up yellow-green purulent sputum for two days. She has had some streaky haemoptysis but is not worried as this has occurred on previous occasions.

Examination

Her observations were stable with a heart rate of 80 per minute and a blood pressure of 124/82. Her respiratory rate was 22 per minute, with reduced air entry bilaterally and diffuse coarse crackles most pronounced over the lower zones posteriorly. Her blood haematology showed a leucocytosis and raised C-reactive protein. Her biochemistry and liver function tests were normal. Chest radiograph and computed tomography (CT) scans were taken (Figures 77.1 and 77.2).

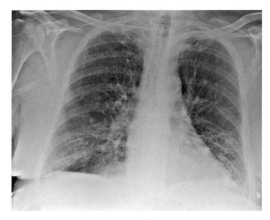

Figure 77.1 Chest radiograph.

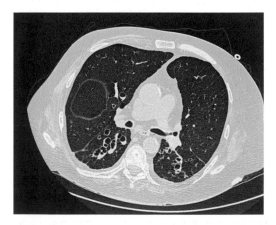

Figure 77.2 Axial CT image taken at the level of the lower lobes.

Question

• What do the chest radiograph and axial CT image demonstrate?

The chest radiograph (Figure 77.1) shows ring opacities (cystic changes) due to the dilatation of bronchi with crowding of the vascular markings and prominent parallel lines (tram tracks) presenting thickened walls of the dilated bronchi.

On the axial CT scan through the lower lobes the bronchi are dilated and larger than the accompanying vessels. This is abnormal and sometimes referred to as the 'signet ring sign'. The signet ring sign consists of a small circle of soft tissue attenuation that abuts a ring of soft tissue attenuation surrounding a larger low attenuating circle of air. The ring of soft tissue attenuation represents the wall of the dilated bronchus seen on an axial CT scan, whereas the low attenuating circle of air represents air within the dilated bronchus. The circle of soft tissue attenuation abutting the ring represents the pulmonary artery that lies adjacent to the dilated bronchus seen in cross-section. In Figure 77.2 dilated, thick-walled, slightly ectatic bronchi are demonstrated within both lower lobes.

Bronchiectasis is the irreversible dilatation of part of the bronchial tree. The bronchi involved are dilated, inflamed and collapsible. This results in airflow obstruction and impaired clearance of secretions. Bronchiectasis is associated with a wide range of disorders, some inherited, such as cystic fibrosis or agammaglobulinaemia, and some acquired, such as necrotizing bacterial infections caused by *Staphylococcus* or *Klebsiella* or early childhood infections caused by measles or *Bordetella pertussis*.

Haemoptysis, as experienced by the patient in this case, is common and may occur in up to 50 per cent of patients. Episodic haemoptysis with little sputum production or 'dry' bronchiectasis is a sequela of tuberculosis. When massive haemoptysis occurs, the bleeding usually originates in dilated bronchial arteries, which contain blood at systemic as opposed to pulmonary pressures.

The diagnosis of bronchiectasis is based on a clinical history of frequent viscid sputum production and characteristic CT scan findings.

Chest radiography is usually the first imaging examination, but the findings are often non-specific and the images may appear normal in patients with minor to moderate disease. Abnormal radiographic findings may be non-specific and confirmation using high-resolution CT (HRCT) scanning may be required.

Although subtle, thick-walled and dilated bronchi are present on the radiograph in Figure 77.1. Potential abnormal plain radiographic findings in bronchiectasis include: parallel line 'tram track' opacities caused by thickened dilated bronchi; ring opacities or cystic spaces as large as 2 cm in diameter resulting from cystic bronchiectasis, sometimes with air–fluid levels; tubular opacities caused by dilated fluid-filled bronchi; increased size and loss of definition of the pulmonary vessels in the affected areas as a result of peri-bronchial fibrosis; crowding of pulmonary vascular markings from the associated loss of volume, usually caused by mucous obstruction of the peripheral bronchi; oligaemia as a result of reduction in pulmonary artery perfusion in severe disease; signs of compensatory hyperinflation of the unaffected lung.

CT, in particular HRCT, scanning has become the imaging modality of choice for demonstrating and defining the extent of bronchiectasis. HRCT allows evaluation of the surrounding lung tissue and assessment for other lesions.

On HRCT scans in patients with bronchiectasis, the internal bronchial diameter may be greater than that of the adjacent artery and there may be a lack of bronchial tapering. The bronchi may be within 1 cm of costal pleura or abut the mediastinal pleura and bronchial wall thickening may be seen. A cystic cluster of thin-walled cystic spaces may be present, often with air–fluid levels.

 KEY POINTS

- Plain chest radiographs are usually the first imaging examination, but the findings are often non-specific and the images may appear normal in patients with minor to moderate disease.
- HRCT scanning is the diagnostic modality of choice and has few limitations.

History

A 65-year-old man presents to his general practitioner (GP) with breathing difficulty over the past month, along with problems chewing, talking and walking up the stairs in his house. Of particular concern, he had noticed his eyelids drooping and he had difficulty maintaining a steady gaze. He noted that he has felt persistently fatigued and his symptoms worsened with activity and improved with rest.

Examination

He was afebrile. His pulse was 74/minute and blood pressure 126/78. The chest was clear, breath sounds vesicular although there was reduced expansion and a respiratory rate of 22/minute.

Neurological examination demonstrated bilateral ptosis along with weakness of the arms, legs and swallowing muscles. The jaw was slack and the voice had a nasal quality. Muscle weakness was worsened by repetitive or sustained use of the muscles involved. Recovery of strength was seen after a period of rest.

Full blood count and biochemistry were normal. Due to the difficulty in breathing, the patient was referred for a chest radiograph (Figure 78.1) and computed tomography (CT) scan (Figure 78.2).

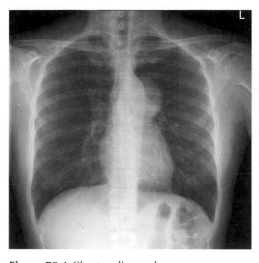
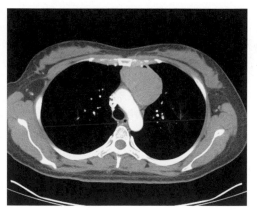

Figure 78.1 Chest radiograph.   **Figure 78.2** CT scan.

Questions

- What is the abnormality on the chest radiograph?
- Where is the lesion anatomically located?
- Does Figure 78.2 confirm your suspicion?
- What is the differential diagnosis?

ANSWER 78

Figure 78.1 shows a smooth, well-defined mass arising from the left side of the mediastinum. By virtue of the fact that the margin of the descending thoracic aorta can be clearly seen, this mass does not lie within the posterior mediastinum. Furthermore, the hilar structures can also be seen making the middle mediastinum an unlikely location. Indeed the axial CT scan seen in Figure 78.2 demonstrates that the mass lies within the anterior mediastinum.

Anatomically the mediastinum lies between the right and left pleura, in and near the median sagittal plane of the chest. It extends from the sternum in front to the vertebral column behind, and contains all the thoracic viscera except the lungs.

It may be divided into superior and inferior parts:

- The superior mediastinum lies above the upper level of the pericardium at the plane drawn from the sternal angle to the disc of T4–T5 (angle of Louis).
- The inferior mediastinum lies below the superior margin of the pericardium and is further subdivided into three parts: anterior – in front of the pericardium; middle – containing the pericardium and its contents; posterior – behind the pericardium.

The mediastinum is surrounded by the chest wall anteriorly, the lungs laterally and the spine posteriorly. It is continuous with the loose connective tissue of the neck, and extends inferiorly onto the diaphragm.

The location of a mass within the mediastinum can be deduced radiologically on the plain chest radiograph by assessing a number of radiological landmarks. In Figure 78.1 the margin of the descending aorta and thoracic vertebrae/ribs, which are posterior mediastinal structures, can be seen crisply and clearly. This suggests that the lesion is not within the posterior mediastinum (where the presence of a mass located in opposition to these structures would cause a silhouette sign). The vascular structures of the hilum are also preserved. Therefore, the mass most likely lies within the anterior compartment. This is confirmed on CT (Figure 78.2).

The anterior mediastinum contains the following structures: thymus, lymph nodes, pulmonary artery, phrenic nerves and thyroid. The most common lesions encountered in the anterior mediastinum arise from thyroid, thymic (thymoma) or lymph node (lymphoma) origin. Germ cell tumours (teratoma) arise from pluripotent cells of the thymus.

This case was later proven to be a thymoma, in the context of myasthenia gravis. Indeed as many as 30–40 per cent of patients who have a thymoma experience symptoms suggestive of myasthenia gravis. The thymus is a lymphoid organ located in the anterior mediastinum. In early life, the thymus is responsible for the development and maturation of cell-mediated immunological functions.

The thymus gland is located behind the sternum in front of the great vessels. It reaches its maximum weight at puberty and undergoes involution thereafter. Peak incidence of thymoma occurs in the fourth to fifth decade of life. No sexual predilection exists.

Of patients with a thymoma, one-third to one-half are asymptomatic. Others often present with local symptoms related to the tumour encroaching on surrounding structures. These patients may present with cough, chest pain, superior vena cava syndrome, dysphagia and hoarseness (if the recurrent laryngeal nerve is involved). One-third of thymoma cases are found on radiographic examinations during a work-up for myasthenia gravis, as in this case.

KEY POINTS

- The anatomical location of a mediastinal mass may be deduced from the plain radiograph by assessing for anatomical landmarks.

History

A 14-year-old girl is thrown from her horse while making a jump. She landed on her head with her neck in the hyperflexed position. She denies any loss of consciousness, although she is taken into accident and emergency with her neck immobilized, complaining of severe pain in her lower cervical spine. She had sustained no other obvious injury and has no significant medical history.

Examination

She is maintaining her airway. Examination of the chest, abdomen and pelvis is unremarkable. Neurological assessment fails to demonstrate a focal deficit. Sensation, power and reflexes are normal in all four limbs. Per rectal examination reveals normal tone.

There is concern regarding her cervical spine injury, therefore a lateral radiograph is performed (Figure 79.1). A computed tomography (CT) scan is subsequently performed with a sagittal reformat image shown in Figure 79.2.

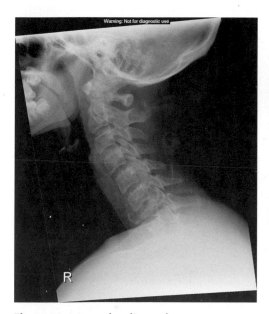

Figure 79.1 Lateral radiograph.

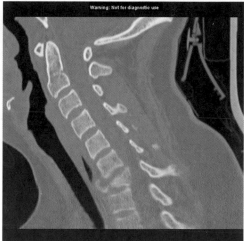

Figure 79.2 Sagittal reformat CT scan.

Questions

- What does the lateral cervical spine radiograph show?
- What does the CT scan demonstrate?

This 14-year-old girl has sustained a hyperflexion 'teardrop' fracture of C7 which is also crushed. There is wedging of the vertebral body with retropulsion of the posterior fragment into the spinal canal. This can be seen on both the initial lateral radiograph Figure 79.1 and more clearly on the sagittal CT image of the cervical spine (Figure 79.2). A flexion teardrop fracture occurs when flexion of the spine, along with vertical axial compression, causes a fracture of the anterior–inferior aspect of the vertebral body. This fragment is displaced anteriorly and resembles a teardrop.

For this fragment to be produced significant posterior ligamentous disruption must occur and as the fragment displaces anteriorly, a significant degree of anterior ligamentous disruption must take place.

This example demonstrates a flexion injury, however, cervical spine injuries are classified according to several other mechanisms of injury in addition to flexion, including flexion–rotation, extension, extension–rotation, vertical compression, lateral flexion and mechanisms resulting in odontoid (C2) fractures and atlanto-occipital dislocation.

The cervical spine should be seen as three distinct columns:

- **Anterior column**: This is composed of the anterior longitudinal ligament and the anterior two-thirds of the vertebral bodies, the annulus fibrosus and the intervertebral discs.
- **Middle column**: This is composed of the posterior longitudinal ligament and the posterior one-third of the vertebral bodies, the annulus and intervertebral discs.
- **Posterior column**: This contains all of the bony elements formed by the pedicles, transverse processes, articulating facets, laminae and spinous processes.

If one column is disrupted, other columns may provide sufficient stability to prevent spinal cord injury. If two columns are disrupted, the spine may move as separate units, increasing the likelihood of spinal cord injury.

This fracture is important to recognize as it is an unstable type of cervical spine fracture involving disruption of all three spinal columns, making this an extremely unstable fracture that frequently is associated with spinal cord injury.

The girl in this case was referred to the spinal service and initially managed with the application of traction with cervical tongs, but later underwent a C7 corpectomy and fusion (Figure 79.3).

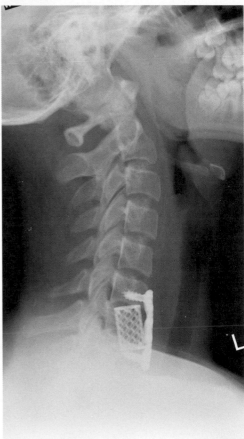

Figure 79.3 Lateral radiograph post surgery showing C7 corpectomy and fusion.

When interpreting lateral cervical views, first you should check the technical adequacy of the radiograph, which must show all seven vertebral bodies *and* the cervicothoracic junction. Next, look for soft tissue changes in predental and prevertebral spaces (if the prevertebral space is widened at any level, a haematoma secondary to a fracture is likely). At the level of C2, prevertebral space should not exceed 7 mm and at the level of C6 and below, where the prevertebral space is widened by the presence of the oesophagus and cricopharyngeal muscle, no more than 22 mm in adults/14 mm in children younger than 15 years.

Then check the alignment of the cervical spine by following three imaginary contour lines:

- The first line connects the anterior margins of all the vertebrae and is referred to as the anterior contour line. It is clearly disrupted in Figure 79.1.
- The second line should connect the posterior aspect of all vertebrae in a similar way and is referred to as the posterior contour line. This is also disrupted in Figure 79.1.
- The third line should connect the bases of the spinous processes. This is referred to as the spinolaminar line.

KEY POINTS

- Approximately 85–90 per cent of cervical spine injuries are evident in lateral view.
- An acceptable lateral view must show all seven vertebral bodies and the cervicothoracic junction.
- It is important to check the alignment of cervical spine by following three imaginary contour lines.
- Soft tissue changes in predental and prevertebral spaces should always be looked for.

History

You are asked to review the abdominal radiograph of a 28-year-old woman who has presented to the accident and emergency department with worsening abdominal pain and diarrhoea. She is known to have a diagnosis of ulcerative colitis and, despite occasional disease exacerbations as a teenager, she has been symptom free for 5 years.

Over the last 2 days she has been complaining of generalized aching abdominal pain. This is associated with diarrhoea that is increasing in frequency and yesterday she opened her bowels nine times. Overnight she was unable to control her loose motions and noticed fresh blood with streaks of pus within the stool. She denies weight loss but gives a history of feeling very lethargic.

She attended the accident and emergency department worried about an acute attack of ulcerative colitis and was found to be tachycardic but normotensive on examination. Her abdomen was distended but not peritonitic, and she reported pain on deep palpation, most marked within the left upper quadrant. Her blood results suggest a degree of renal impairment and dehydration, with a slightly elevated white cell count but normal haemoglobin.

Examination

As part of the initial investigations an abdominal radiograph was performed (Figure 80.1).

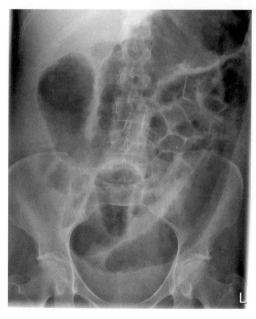

Figure 80.1 Abdominal radiograph.

Questions

- What does the abdominal radiograph demonstrate?
- What further imaging is recommended?
- Is there a differential diagnosis for these appearances?

ANSWER 80

This is an anterior–posterior abdominal radiograph of an adult female. There is gross abnormality of the large bowel with widespread dilatation most marked at the splenic flexure, where the maximal bowel diameter measures 10.3 cm (normal large bowel diameter <6 cm). There is abnormal thickening and 'thumbprinting' of the colonic wall with loss of normal haustrations due to mucosal oedema. There is no evidence of small bowel involvement and no characteristic appearances of 'Rigler's sign' (see below) to suggest extraluminal free gas related to bowel perforation. The appearances are consistent with colitis with bowel dilatation, in keeping with toxic megacolon. Urgent surgical opinion should be sought and clinical correlation advised since perforation is a significant risk.

A computed tomography (CT) scan of the abdomen and pelvis is recommended to characterize the radiograph findings further (Figure 80.2). Ideally, this should be performed with intravenous contrast in the portal venous phase, however, renal function derangement from fluid sequestration may make this impossible. The possible need for surgery is a relative contraindication to oral contrast enhancement.

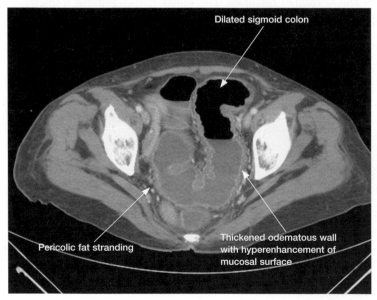

Figure 80.2 Enhanced CT scan.

This single enhanced CT image acquired at a level just superior to the femoral acetabulae demonstrates dilatation and thickening of the sigmoid colon. There is hyperenhancement of the mucosa and muscularis propria, which outline an iso-attenuating oedematous submucosa. There is associated pericolic fat stranding. These findings suggest acute inflammatory change. There is no evidence of free fluid within the pelvis and no extraluminal free gas on this image, although the whole study should be reviewed to exclude perforation.

Inflammation of the colon is termed 'colitis' and its causes are numerous:

• **Infection:** bacteria (*E. coli*, *Salmonella*), parasites (amoebiasis), fungi (histoplasmosis) and viruses (HIV, CMV) can all cause pancolitis and marked wall oedema.

- **Ischaemia:** The splenic flexure/descending colon are a watershed area demarcated by the blood supply from the superior and inferior mesenteric arteries. It is particularly susceptible to ischaemia of any cause (e.g. atherosclerosis), and the colitic appearances can mimic inflammatory bowel disease. The characteristic appearance of air within the wall of the colon is termed 'pneumatosis coli' and is highly suggestive of ischaemic colitis. It is usually a premorbid phenomenon (Figure 80.3).

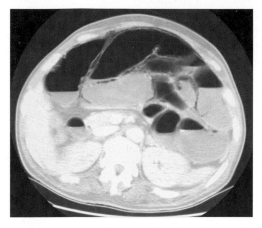

Figure 80.3 Scan showing air within the wall of the colon: pneumotosis coli.

- **Pseudomembranous:** Often caused by an overgrowth of the *Clostridium difficile* bacterium related to antibiotic usage, predisposed patients can suffer a pancolitis with deterioration to toxic megacolon.
- **Inflammatory bowel disease:** Ulcerative colitis (UC) and Crohn's disease are difficult to differentiate by history alone and require histological characterization. Radiologically, UC is often left sided with shallow mucosal ulcers extending down to the rectum with small bowel sparing. Crohn's is a discontinuous, full thickness disease, often with deep penetrating ulcers sparing the rectum and commonly seen at the terminal ileum.
- **Toxic megacolon:** This can occur in any form of colitis, but is particularly prevalent in UC. Uncontrolled fulminant colitis can lead to transmural involvement with rapid dilatation of the large bowel. There are large fluid shifts and the patient is often toxic and shocked. As a surgical emergency, it requires rapid identification and carries a significant risk of mortality.

Named after Leo George Rigler, an American radiologist, the eponym 'Rigler's sign' was derived from his paper entitled 'Spontaneous pneumoperitoneum: a roentgenologic sign found in the supine position'.[1] Until 1941, the only documented sign of intraperitoneal free gas was seeing crescenteric gas contrasted against the diaphragm and solid abdominal viscera on erect chest radiographs. Rigler described that is it possible to 'observe both the contour of the inner and outer wall of the bowel'[1] in supine positioning when there is significant intraperitoneal free gas. This is also known as the 'double wall sign', and is an abnormal finding unless the patient has undergone recent surgery or laparoscopy (Figure 80.4).

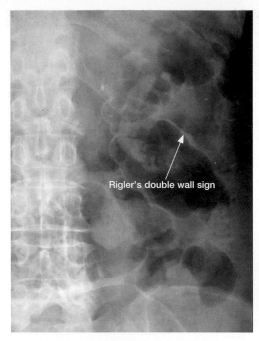

Rigler's double wall sign

Figure 80.4 Radiograph showing Rigler's sign.

 KEY POINTS

- The bowel is said to be dilated when the cross-sectional diameter exceeds 3 cm for small bowel and 6 cm for large bowel.
- Pneumatosis coli is highly suggestive of ischaemic colitis and carries high mortality.
- 'Rigler's sign' is pathognomonic for the diagnosis of intraperitoneal free gas.

Reference

1. Rigler, L.G. (1941) Spontaneous pneumoperitoneum: a roentgenologic sign found in the supine position. *Radiology* 37: 604–607.

History

A 65-year-old woman attends her local accident and emergency department following a mechanical fall. While walking her dog this morning, she slipped on the icy pavement and fell forward, putting out her left hand to break her fall. She heard a 'crack' and had an instant sharp stabbing pain in her left wrist. Noticing an obvious deformity and experiencing severe pain on all movements, she called her husband who collected her and bought her to hospital.

She has a history of gallstone disease and a cholecystectomy. She went through the menopause aged 55 years, and was on hormone replacement therapy for the following 6 years. She has never had a bone density scan or suffered any previous fractures. She takes no regular medication and has never taken corticosteroids.

Examination

The triage nurse has requested a wrist X-ray (Figure 81.1).

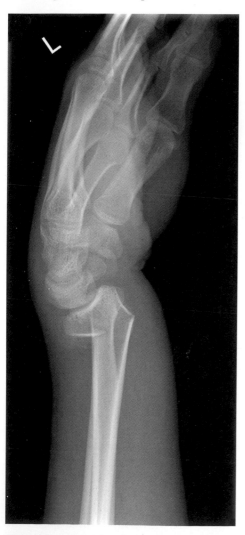

Questions
- What does this X-ray show?
- What is the common mechanism of injury and how is it treated?

Figure 81.1 Lateral radiograph of the left wrist.

Figure 81.1 is a lateral radiograph of the left wrist in an adult patient. There is abnormality seen in the distal radius with interruption of the normal smooth cortical line, and a linear cortical breach extending horizontally through the distal radius. There is loss of normal alignment with the distal radius fragment dorsally angulated by approximately 30 degrees. The radiocarpal joint is not involved but the carpal bones are displaced posteriorly with associated overlying soft tissue swelling. It is normal practice to look at the wrist in two views.

This anterior–posterior (AP) view of the same patient (Figure 81.2) confirms a comminuted fracture of the distal radius with dorsal angulation of the distal fragment. There is also a fracture of the ulna styloid with medial displacement of the distal fragment associated with soft tissue swelling. No other bony injury is seen, most importantly to the scaphoid. There is no radiographic evidence of scapholunate dislocation. These features are in keeping with a complex Colles' fracture to the left wrist.

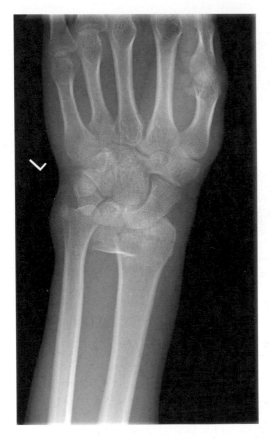

Figure 81.2 AP radiograph view of the left wrist.

This type of wrist fracture is named after Abraham Colles, an Irish surgeon from Dublin (1773–1843). A Colles' fracture is the commonest fracture to the forearm and is usually sustained from a mechanical fall. The patient uses an outstretched hand to break the fall, with the radius fracturing horizontally approximately 2 cm from the articulating surface. The patient's bodyweight forces the distal fracture fragment dorsally and commonly fractures the ulna styloid in the process. The nature of the injury predisposes the osteoporotic elderly and active young patients (skateboarders, snowboarders) to this type of fracture. Reduction of the fracture is essential to reduce the long-term risks of fused misalignment, deformity, reduced range of movement and joint osteoarthritis. This is most commonly done in the accident and emergency department under sedation and local anaesthetic (Bier's block). The wrist is reduced and temporarily placed in a cast, held in palmar flexion with ulna deviation to maintain the reduction. Orthopaedic assessment in the fracture clinic may leave undisplaced fractures in a cast with no further treatment, however significant deformity usually requires surgical fixation, taking into account age, hand dominance, occupation, radial variance, intra-articular extension and dorsal tilt (>20 degrees).

The four commonest adult wrist fractures to recognize are shown in Figure 81.3.

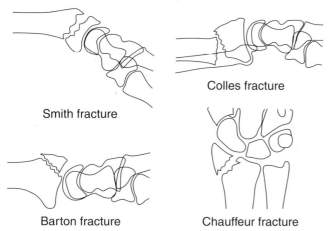

Smith fracture

Colles fracture

Barton fracture

Chauffeur fracture

Figure 81.3 Adult wrist fractures. Reproduced from Reference 1 with permission.

In addition to Colles' fracture, these include:

- **Smith fracture:** Commonly called the reverse Colles' fracture, this is commonly seen in older osteoporotic patients who fall onto a clenched fist. A horizontal fracture to the distal radius is sustained with volar angulation of the distal fragment.
- **Barton fracture:** This injury, also sustained by falling on an outstretched hand, fractures the radial head vertically with dorsal angulation to the distal fragment. This has intra-articular extension and is associated with carpal dislocation.
- **Chauffeur fracture:** Sudden ulnar deviation and dorsiflexion causes an avulsion fracture to the radial styloid with lateral displacement of the fracture fragment. Associated with lunate dislocation, these fractures were commonly sustained by chauffeurs when an automobile backfired during a hand crank start.

 KEY POINTS

- A Colles' fracture is the commonest fracture of the forearm and is usually sustained by falling on an outstretched hand.
- Fracture reduction is essential to reduce the risk of long-term osteoarthritis.
- Fracture clinic assessment is integral in the follow-up of all fractures.

Reference

1. Dahnert, W. (2011) *Radiology Review Manual*, 7th edn. Philadelphia: Lippincott Williams and Wilkins.

CASE 82: A KNOWN CASE OF INFLAMMATORY BOWEL DISEASE

History

A barium follow-through study has been requested on a 22-year-old woman who has a history of Crohn's disease. She presented 2 days earlier with abdominal pain localized to the left lower quadrant and occasional diarrhoea. She denies vomiting and is still passing flatus freely. Despite taking her Crohn's medication regularly, she feels this is an acute flare-up of her disease and sought medical attention.

Examination

Examination reveals a patient who is comfortable at rest with normal observations. Her abdomen is generally soft on palpation but there is local guarding and tenderness in the left iliac fossa. Per rectal examination does not demonstrate rectal blood.

Investigations show an elevated white cell count (90 per cent neutrophils) with normal renal and liver function tests. Her C-reactive protein is 160 mg/L.

An abdominal radiograph did not demonstrate bowel obstruction and a barium follow-through study is requested to assess her bowel mucosa and look for fibrotic strictures (Figure 82.1).

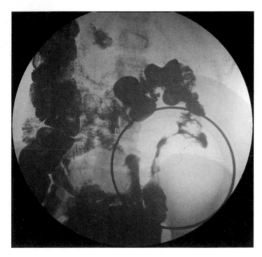

Figure 82.1 Barium follow-though.

Questions

- How is this procedure performed and what does it demonstrate?
- What other imaging modalities are used to diagnose and follow-up patients with Crohn's disease?
- What are the extra-intestinal manifestations of Crohn's disease?

This is a single image of a barium follow-though study, acquired with the patient in a prone position and centred on the right lower quadrant. There is good opacification of the small bowel, and contrast appears to have passed freely into the large bowel with opacification of the descending colon. This image demonstrates a 25cm stricture of the terminal ileum, with the adjacent caecal pole also appearing abnormal and oedematous. There is small bowel loop separation in the right lower quadrant, probably related to lymphoedema of the bowel wall and adjacent fibrofatty proliferation, however an inflammatory mass lesion (e.g. abscess) needs to be excluded. There is no prestenotic dilation and the appearance of the remaining small bowel is normal. The findings are in keeping with active inflammatory stricture related to Crohn's disease, and a computed tomography (CT) abdomen and pelvis is recommended to exclude a drainable collection.

Local hospital policy dictates the exact procedural technique of a barium follow-through study: a patient is required to drink a set volume of radio-opaque barium, often diluted with water and mixed with a prokinetic agent (e.g. metoclopramide) to promote rapid transit through the bowel. The barium is screened though the small bowel under fluoroscopy, and sequential images are obtained at different points in time. The patient is often imaged in the prone position to splay the bowel loops and reduce composite shadowing from overlying loops of bowel. Focal compression can improve visualization as demonstrated in this image, with the compression paddle highlighting the area of tapered narrowing at the terminal ileum.

As well as small bowel follow-through studies, there is also a role for both CT and magnetic resonance imaging (MRI). A CT scan is quick to perform and usually accessible 24 hours per day, but it carries a significant radiation exposure and Crohn's patients are often young. CT is employed in the acute setting to characterize the extent of acute inflammation and also to exclude abscess formation (Figure 82.2).

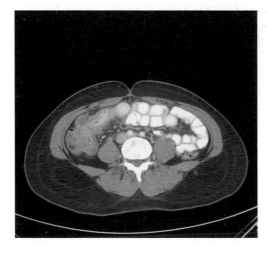

Figure 82.2 Axial CT scan.

A CT scan of the same patient, acquired at the level of the terminal ileum following intravenous and oral contrast administration was performed. It confirms an acute inflammatory reaction centred on the terminal ileum and caecal pole with bowel wall thickening, mucosal hyperenhancement and perinephric fat stranding with small volume pericolic lymph nodes seen. There is no evidence of an inflammatory mass lesion or drainable collection.

MRI is preferable for the long-term follow-up of Crohn's disease patients, and has a high sensitivity for disease evaluation without exposing the patient to ionizing radiation. MRI has good soft tissue contrast and provides further information to differentiate between fibrosis and inflammation.[1] This can dictate whether a patient continues medical treatment or requires surgery. However, MRI is expensive and time consuming to perform and does not provide accurate mucosal detail obtained in a follow-through study.

Figure 82.3 is a single image from an MRI half Fourier acquisition single shot turbo spin echo (HASTE) sequence of the same patient taken 6 months later, and demonstrates a fibrotic stricture of the terminal ileum measuring approximately 6 cm, with no evidence of active inflammation.

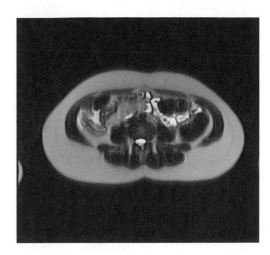

Figure 82.3 Axial MRI image from HASTE sequence.

Crohn's disease is an inflammatory condition that can affect the bowel anywhere from the mouth to the anus. Gastrointestinal symptoms include diarrhoea, rectal bleeding, malabsorption and abdominal pain. Patients suffer from bowel strictures causing obstruction, adhesion formation and fistulation, often resulting in surgery. As well as an increased risk of malignancy, patients have a range of extraintestinal manifestations (Table 82.1).

Table 82.1 Extraintestinal manifestations of Crohn's disease

Hepatobiliary	Fatty liver
	Gallstone disease
	Pancreatitis
Genitourinary	Urolithiasis
	Renal amyloidosis
Musculoskeletal	Clubbing
	Hypertropthic osteoarthropathy
	Avascular necrosis
Erythema nodosum	
Uveitis	
Growth retardation (childhood onset)	

References

1. Lawrance, I.C., Welman, C.J., Shipman, P. and Murray, K. (2009) Correlation of MRI-determined small bowel Crohn's disease categories with medical response and surgical pathology. *World Journal of Gastroenterology* 15: 3367–75.

History

A 44-year-old woman attends the accident and emergency department with a painful leg. She is a tourist on holiday, and flew in from New Zealand on a 23-hour flight arriving 2 days ago. Since landing in the UK, her left leg has developed an achy pain with associated swelling and erythema. It has become increasingly difficult to walk, and despite analgesia with elevation of the leg her symptoms have not resolved. She is alarmed by the swelling and attended hospital with near complete immobility due to the pain.

She is normally a fit and healthy individual with no significant medical history. Apart from occasional homeopathic remedies for insomnia, she is taking no regular prescribed medication other than the oral contraceptive pill.

Examination

On examination there is swelling of the left ankle, calf and thigh with marked tenderness in the calf muscles and some tenderness medially in the thigh. There is some redness of the leg. There is no knee joint effusion and peripheral pulses are present.

As part of her investigations, a lower limb ultrasound is organized with the radiology department (Figure 83.1).

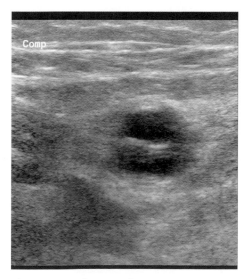

Figure 83.1 Ultrasound.

Questions
- What does this ultrasound image demonstrate?
- How does ultrasound work?
- What are the strengths and limitations of ultrasound?

This static image is a cross-sectional view of the superficial femoral vein (SFV) lying adjacent to the superficial femoral artery (Figure 83.2). Fluid on ultrasound is normally hypoechoic in appearance as demonstrated by the flowing blood within the femoral artery. The intraluminal appearances of the adjacent vein are not anechoic, and return a heterogeneous echogenic signal. Subsequent images demonstrate non-compressibility of this SFV in keeping with a solid intraluminal venous component.

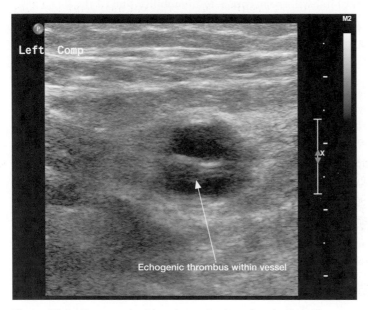

Figure 83.2 Ultrasound with echogenic thrombus indicated.

Figure 83.3 shows a longitudinal Doppler image of the same region with flow demonstrated within the femoral artery. The SFV again demonstrates an ill-defined heterogeneous echogenic appearance, and only a trace of flow is demonstrated.

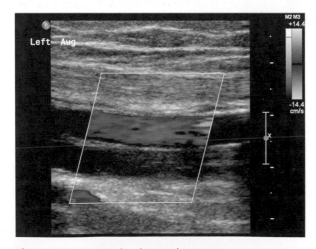

Figure 83.3 Longitudinal Doppler image.

In summary, there is echogenic thrombus seen within the left SFV with reduced patency, compressibility and flow in keeping with a deep vein thrombosis (DVT). The possible complications are pulmonary embolism and post-phlebitic problems in the limb. Anticoagulation is indicated. The risk factors in this case are the long flight and the oral contraceptive pill. The oral contraceptive pill should be stopped, with appropriate contraceptive advice, and anticoagulation would normally be continued for 6 months with a first thrombus and an identified precipitant.

Ultrasound is the use of sound waves to image the human body. The sound waves are of such high frequency that they are inaudible to the human ear (e.g. 2–20 MHz). An ultrasound probe is designed to convert an electrical signal into acoustic energy and does so by utilizing the unique properties of piezoelectric crystals (most commonly microcrystalline lead zirconate titanate (PZT)). The ultrasound probe comprises a compressed layer of PZT, which is coated in silver to allow electrical conduction. Passing an alternating electrical current causes the PZT to expand and contract with the production of a sinusoidal sound wave of a particular frequency and wavelength. The shape of the ultrasound probe and a rubber-coated window can focus the sound wave, allowing an operator to control its direction.

The sound waves do not pass through the body freely, and tissues of differing density cause the beam to be reflected back towards the probe. The degree of sound wave transmission through a tissue before it is reflected is dictated by the acoustic impedance of the tissue through which it is passing. Subtle density changes (e.g. within soft tissue) cause the reflected 'echoes' to return to the probe at different times. The returning sinusoidal sound wave compresses the PZT, which converts the acoustic echo back into electrical energy and allows complex computer programs to form a picture on the operator's screen. When there is a sudden density change (e.g. muscle to bone/muscle to gas) the majority of the sound wave is either transmitted or reflected and no images beyond this density interface can be generated. This limits the use of ultrasound in imaging the lungs or deep to bone.

Each probe has a fixed frequency, with a higher frequency returning more echoes over a period of time and forming an image of superior resolution compared to probes of a lower frequency. Unfortunately, the acoustic impedance of higher frequency and shorter wavelength sound waves, limits the depth they can travel. Higher frequencies are therefore recommended for the imaging of superficial pathology (e.g. a subcutaneous lump), while deeper imaging (e.g. abdomen) requires a probe of increased wavelength, and the reduced frequency allows only for an image of reduced resolution. As with many other aspects of radiology (e.g. CT dose versus noise), image resolution and depth penetration is a trade-off.

As an imaging modality that does not involve the use of ionizing radiation, ultrasound is preferred, if appropriate, to CT or X-ray. Some of the strengths and weaknesses of ultrasound are listed in Table 83.1.

Table 83.1 Strengths and weaknesses of ultrasound

Strengths	Weaknesses
• No ionizing radiation: This is especially important in the young people and pregnant women	• Operator dependent: Experience may dictate a more accurate report
• Cheap: Compared to a CT or MRI scanner, ultrasound machines are inexpensive	• Body habitus: It is more difficult to generate a diagnostic image in larger people
• Readily available: No patient preparation or other healthcare professionals required	• Density changes: Images are limited by bone, bowel gas and normal aerated lung
• Real time: Allows for functional imaging (e.g. contrast enhancement) and needle guidance for biopsy procedures	
• Portable: Ultrasound machines can be taken to immobile patients (e.g. ITU)	

KEY POINTS

- Ultrasound has a high sensitivity for the diagnosis of a DVT and carries no risk of ionizing radiation exposure to the patient.
- Ultrasound assesses compressibility, patency and flow of the deep venous system.
- The major limitations of ultrasound are operator dependence and patient body habitus.

History

A 14-year-old boy is referred to the interventional radiology department following an ear, nose and throat (ENT) multidisciplinary meeting (MDM). He complains of a 6-week history of epistaxis that has been increasing in frequency, currently with approximately eight episodes of bleeding per day. No predisposing factors are to be found on history and the spontaneous bleeds can occur at any time. The worst bleeds are at night and he recently reports a single episode when he woke from sleep feeling as though he was choking from a spontaneous episode of bleeding. At that time the bleeding lasted more than 30 minutes and required hospital attendance for nasal packing. He has never needed a blood transfusion.

Examination

On review by the ENT registrar on call at the accident and emergency department, initial screening bloods were unremarkable but the patient was kept in hospital overnight for observation. The next morning the nasal packing was removed and direct visualization with a flexible nasendoscope revealed an area of friable soft tissue abnormality on the right side. The patient was referred for a contrast-enhanced computed tomography (CT) scan, which revealed an avidly arterially enhancing soft tissue mass in the post-nasal space with extension into the retroantral region. The pterygopalatine fossa was widened and a diagnosis of juvenile angiofibroma was made with supply from the right spheno-palatine artery. The patient was discussed at the ENT MDM and referred for embolization under the interventional radiologists (Figure 84.1).

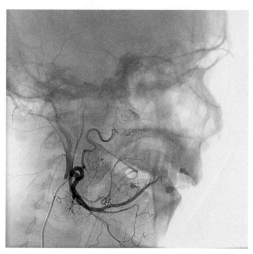

Figure 84.1 Digital subtraction angiography.

Questions

- How was this procedure performed?
- How are catheters and sheaths sized?
- What embolization materials are available?

This case is designed to inform the reader of a few of the devices that are available to an interventional radiologist and the application of them. It also highlights the importance of having a good understanding of vascular anatomy and patient preparation.

The patient was admitted electively to the paediatric ward and the case performed under general anaesthesia. The right common femoral artery was punctured under ultrasound guidance with local anaesthetic cover by a micro-puncture needle. A 0.018″ Mandrel was passed into the common iliac artery and a 4 French (Fr) sheath was inserted at the puncture site. A 0.035″ standard wire was passed into the aortic arch over which was passed a directional catheter. The wire was exchanged for a 0.035″ hydrophilic angled wire and the catheter/wire combination was used to selectively cannulate first the brachiocephalic trunk followed by the common carotid and external carotid arteries. A selective hand-injected angiogram was performed to characterize the vascular anatomy (Figure 84.2).

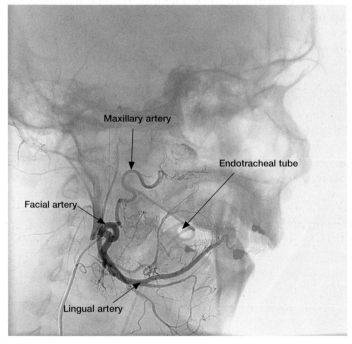

Maxillary artery

Endotracheal tube

Facial artery

Lingual artery

Figure 84.2

Having achieved a stable position with the guide catheter, a 2.8 Fr microcatheter set was used to cannulate the right maxillary artery and advance it for selective cannulation of the sphenopalatine artery. Position was confirmed with angiography and embolization was performed with 500–700 μm polyvinyl acetate (PVA) particles until haemostasis was achieved. There were no unexpected complications and post procedure the patient was cared for by ENT with a successful outcome and no further epistaxis reported.

Catheters and sheaths (Figure 84.3) are the basic tools of an interventional radiologist, and a good understanding of how their size is measured is essential for effective use of a catheter/sheath combination. A sheath is used to secure vascular access and provide stability for the safe passage and manipulation of a catheter through it. They are sized

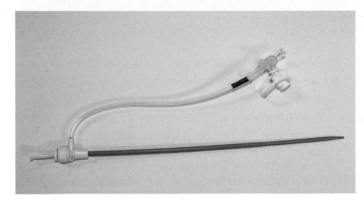

Figure 84.3

according to the French gauge system (Fr) where 1 Fr is 0.33 mm. The bigger the French size the larger the diameter, and this is not to be confused with the needle gauge system where the diameter of a needle is 1/gauge (therefore the larger the gauge the smaller the needle). The French size of a catheter refers to its outer diameter, while when referring to a sheath the French size corresponds to its inner diameter. Therefore a 4 Fr catheter will pass through a 4 Fr sheath.

Embolization procedures are minimally invasive and use the vascular channels of the body to deliver a particular agent to the site of pathology. There are many embolization products on the market, and the most appropriate one is selected depending on the outcome that needs to be achieved. They can be either permanent or temporary but are grossly classified into four categories:

- **Liquid agents:** This is a form of liquid glue that can be injected via a catheter to flow through complex vascular anatomy and solidify, thereby reducing arterial or venous blood flow. They are commonly used in the treatment of arterio-venous malformations (AVMs).
- **Particle agents:** This type of embolization material is used in small arteries or pre-capillary arterioles. They come in a range of sizes (approximately 50–1200 μm) and are predominantly permanent. They have both a mechanical property and clump together to reduce blood flow, but also deliberately induce inflammation to promote clotting. The major disadvantage is that they carry a risk of unwanted distal embolization if not targeted specifically within the blood vessel of choice.
- **Coils:** These are lengths of platinum or stainless steel that are extruded out of a catheter into a high-flowing blood vessel. They are designed to deliberately coil within the vessel and often carry Dacron wool feathers, which slow blood flow causing a mechanical clot and haemostasis. It is a form of permanent embolization and is commonly used in AVMs, testicular vein embolization and in uncontrolled haemorrhage.
- **Plugs:** This is a form of permanent embolization. The plug is appropriately selected for size and then delivered to a vessel through a catheter in a collapsed form. Its delivery can be highly accurate and it is re-expanded within the vessel before detachment to cause a mechanical embolization.

 KEY POINTS

- Optimal patient preparation and procedural planning is of paramount importance in any interventional procedure.
- An excellent understanding of expected and aberrant anatomy is essential.
- In the French gauge system, 1 Fr is equivalent to 0.33 mm in diameter.

History

A 44-year-old Afro-Caribbean woman has been referred for assessment. She complains of gradual abdominal distension over the last few years. Until recently this was not associated with abdominal pain outside of her normal menstrual periods, but over the last month she has had a constant achy pain in her stomach. She denies any chance of pregnancy and reports no change in her bowel habit. She has been gaining weight over the last few years despite activity and dieting.

Examination

Examination reveals a distended but soft abdomen, with a fullness centrally that is tender on deep palpation. This has clear examination margins unrelated to other abdominal viscera and does not move on respiration. Haematinic studies reveal a slight microcytic anaemia with normal renal, thyroid and liver function parameters.

An abdominal ultrasound study organized by her general practitioner (GP) had demonstrated the presence of a large soft tissue/cystic mass extending up from her pelvis. The patient was referred following an magnetic resonance imaging (MRI) study (Figure 85.1).

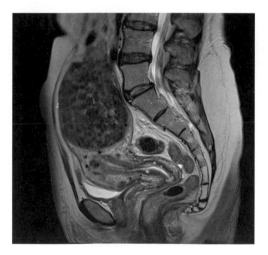

Figure 85.1 Sagittal T2-weighted MRI scan.

Questions

- What is this examination and what is the main abnormality?
- Can you classify the type of abnormality seen?
- How are these lesions normally diagnosed and treated?

ANSWER 85

Figure 85.1 is a T2-weighted image of the pelvis from an MRI study acquired in the sagittal plane. There is a broad-based pedunculated lesion arising from the uterine fundus. This measures approximately 14.5×8.4cm in maximal dimensions and is of predominantly low signal intensity. Subsequent post-gadolinium imaging demonstrated avid enhancement. When comparing it to neighbouring tissue types, the lesion has slightly lower signal characteristics to the adjacent myometrium of the uterus, confirming the diagnosis of a subserosal fibroid. A prominent leash of blood vessels around the right side of the fibroid appears to feed the fibroid. The fibroid also contains a well-defined unilocular central cystic component measuring 9.6×7.0cm. The fluid within the cystic component is hyperintense on T1-weighted images, in keeping with haemorrhagic degeneration. The cystic component does not demonstrate any vascularity.

Uterine fibroids result from benign proliferation of the smooth muscle of the myometrium, and can therefore interchangeably be referred to as uterine leiomyomas. They are the commonest gynaecological malignancy, and have an increased incidence in Afro-Caribbean people with approximately 50 per cent of all women affected.[1]

Dependent on oestrogen for growth, it is unusual for women to be diagnosed with fibroid disease in the post-menopausal period or before the age of 30 years, with the exception of younger pregnant women where changes in the oestrogen : progesterone ratio can see rapid fibroid growth in the first trimester. Fibroid size and multiplicity can vary, with the commonest symptoms being pelvic pain, abdominal distension, dysmenorrhoea and menorrhagia. Fibroids large enough to distort the uterine cavity can be responsible for infertility or miscarriage, and can also cause urinary frequency when pressing on the bladder anteriorly. As a highly vascular tumour, if the fibroid size is such that it outgrows its own blood supply, myxoid or haemorrhagic degeneration can occur as seen in Figure 85.2.

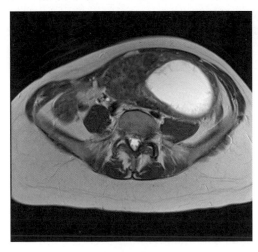

Figure 85.2 Axial T2-weighted MRI scan.

Their position in relation to the wall of the uterus allows for classification:

- **Submucosal:** Growth centred on the inner myometrium allows fibroids to project into the uterine cavity.
- **Intramural:** The commonest subtype, with most patients remaining asymptomatic.
- **Subserosal:** Centred on the outer myometrium, these fibroids are exophytic and can be pedunculated with increased risk of torsion or infarction.

The differential diagnoses associated with the symptoms of fibroid disease are wide, and imaging is essential. Radiologists would advocate the use of ultrasound in the first instance, as this is quick and easily accessible, with no radiation dose to the patient. Optimal views of the uterus would be achieved with a transvaginal scan, although good views of the uterus can be obtained transabdominally, ideally with a full bladder. The role of computed tomography (CT) is limited and there is a significant radiation dose to the radiosensitve pelvic organs.

On ultrasound, fibroids are usually seen as ill-defined rounded hypoechoic heterogeneous lesions associated with distorted uterine architecture. The fibroids have similar ultrasound appearances to the adjacent myometrium, and echogenic bands separating bundles of smooth muscle can be delineated. The presence of calcification is common, demonstrated by echobright foci within the fibroid with posterior acoustic shadowing. Doppler assessment can demonstrate avid vascularity.

MRI is the gold standard imaging modality for accurate fibroid characterization. It can provide clear zonal anatomy for surgical planning and reliably exclude cystic or haemorrhagic degeneration. Imaging sequences of MRI are out of the remit of this case and fibroids can have a variety of appearances, however, fibroids are classically of low signal on T2-weighted images and iso- or hypo-intense to myometrium on T1-weighted images. Calcium would appear low signal on all sequences, with fibroid degeneration appearing as high signal on T2. The degree of haemorrhage, myxoid or cystic degeneration can be variable and is best reviewed on T1 for characterization.

Until the mid 1990s, the only treatment available for symptomatic fibroid disease was surgery in the form of myomectomy or hysterectomy. These procedures carry significant morbidity and require an inpatient stay. As an alternative, interventional radiologists can now offer uterine artery embolization (UAE) to appropriate patients. This is a minimally invasive technique, with selective cannulation of both uterine arteries via a percutaneous groin puncture of the external iliac artery. Under direct fluoroscopic vision, embolization material is instilled to selectively thrombose the uterine artery and deliberately infarct the fibroid. This reduces tumour volume and improves patient symptoms over time, hopefully avoiding the need for aggressive surgery.

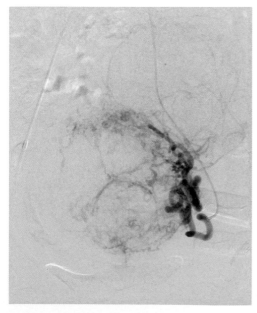

Figure 85.3 Uterine embolization.

KEY POINTS

- MRI is the gold standard examination for the assessment of uterine fibroid disease.
- Fibroid position in relation to the wall of the uterus allows for classification.
- Uterine artery embolization is a minimally invasive treatment option for fibroid disease.

References

1. Dahnert, W. (2007) *Radiology Review Manual*, 6th edn. Philadelphia: Lippincott Williams and Wilkins.

History

A 35-year-old man is sent to the accident and emergency department by his general practitioner (GP) after complaining of shortness of breath. The symptoms started 10 days ago with a chesty cough, which has become productive of yellow/brown sputum over the last week. He has also noticed increasing shortness of breath and reports a reducing exercise tolerance to less than two flights of stairs. He is a smoker of 10 cigarettes per week, with no relevant past medical or drug history.

On visiting the GP last week, some inspiratory crackles were heard on auscultation in the left mid zone, and a diagnosis of a respiratory tract infection was made. He was pre-scribed a course of amoxicillin but his symptoms have not resolved. He attended the GP today for follow-up and was referred to the accident and emergency department.

Examination

On examination he appears short of breath at rest with use of accessory muscles. His temperature is 38.6°C and he complains of left-sided chest pain on deep breathing. Auscultation reveals coarse crackles in the left mid zone. A sputum sample is green and blood stained. A chest radiograph has been arranged for further assessment (Figure 86.1).

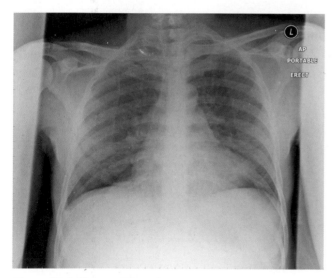

Figure 86.1 Chest radiograph.

Questions

- What does the radiograph show and in which lobe is the pathology?
- Should we worry about the risk of radiation exposure if this patient needs follow-up X-rays?
- Which radiological examinations carry the largest radiation exposure?

Figure 86.1 is an anterior–posterior (AP) chest radiograph of an adult male patient taken in the erect position. It is adequately penetrated but slightly rotated to the right. There is a patchy area of airspace opacification within the left lower zone that lies adjacent to the left heart border obscuring the normal cardiomediastinal contour. Air bronchograms are demonstrated in keeping with consolidation. They are caused by opacification of the lung tissue around air-containing airways. The presence of a 'silhouette sign' and obscuration of one part of the cardiomediastinal border can accurately localize the lung pathology to a particular lobe. In a two-dimensional radiograph a cardiomediastinal border will be lost when up against consolidated lung, but maintained when still lying adjacent to air-containing lung. This is termed the 'silhouette sign'. In this case, loss of the left heart border with preservation of the hemidiaphragm is in keeping with the silhouette sign of lingular consolidation. An annotated chest radiograph demonstrating the normal cardio-mediastinal borders is shown in Figure 86.2.

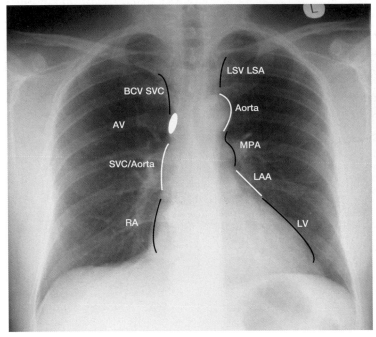

LSV = left subclavian vein
LSA = left subclavian artery
BCV = brachiocephalic vein
SCV = superior vena cava
AV = atrioventricular node
RA = right atrium
LAA = left atrial appendage
LV = left ventricle
MPA = main pulmonary artery

Figure 86.2 Chest radiograph with borders annotated.

For lingular consolidation amoxicillin would not be the appropriate antibiotic and following adequate treatment, if the radiograph changes fail to resolve, further investigations to rule out an obstructive lesion might be indicated.

Several different types of radiation are used in diagnostic imaging, but the principal radiation source, and the one that a patient is regularly exposed to, is X-rays. There is an understandable inherent fear of radiation exposure, but the risks associated with radiation exposure are only realized when there is absorption of energy by living tissue. High-energy beams that pass straight through a person with no absorption are harmless, but absorption causes free radical formation which directly damages cell DNA/RNA, leading to cell death or transformation. Unfortunately, it is the absorption characteristics in human tissues of differing densities that allow a diagnostic picture to be produced. The use of ionizing radiation is therefore strictly controlled through government regulations, most notably the Ionising Radiation (and Medial Exposure) Regulations (IRMER) 2000.

The effects of radiation can be seen either in the exposed individual (somatic effects) or may be realized in the offspring of an exposed individual. These types of effects are termed hereditary and can be either deterministic or stochastic:

- **Deterministic:** Effects of radiation exposure are only seen when the amount of radiation a patient is exposed to exceeds a certain level. Beyond this threshold, the likelihood of detrimental effects rapidly increases, but below it, no risk is inferred.
- **Stochastic:** These effects do not recognize a threshold dose, with the risks of cancers and genetic abnormalities sharing a linear relationship with the degree of exposure: the greater the exposure, the greater the risk.

The types of abnormality seen depend on the type of tissue exposed, with some organs of the body being more radiosensitive than others, for example, the reproductive organs or lens of the eye. It is also important to recognize that we are inherently exposed to natural radiation every day, mainly from cosmic rays and radon decay. The average dose to the UK population per year from these natural sources is approximately 2.2 mSv. Some areas of the United Kingdom have higher exposure (e.g. 7 mSv in Cornwall) from local geographical factors. We can use these figures as a benchmark to help assess the risk of radiation exposure from diagnostic imaging when ordering an X-ray or computed tomography (CT) scan. If the option of an imaging modality that does not expose the patient to ionizing radiation is available and appropriate (e.g. magnetic resonance or ultrasound), then this should be considered in the first instance. Radiation exposures are listed in Table 86.1.

Table 86.1 Radiation exposures from various imaging modalities

Examination	Dose (mSv)	Equivalent number of chest X-rays	Equivalent amount of natural radiation
Chest X-ray	0.02	1	3 days
Skull X-ray	0.06	3	9 days
Lumbar spine X-ray	1	50	5 months
Abdomen X-ray	0.7	35	4 months
Barium enema	7.2	360	3.2 years
CT head	2	100	10 months
CT chest	8	400	3.6 years
CT abdo/pelvis	10	500	4.5 years
V/Q scan	1	50	6 months

By thinking in terms of the number of equivalent chest X-rays a patient is exposed to during a single study, a doctor can gauge the risk/benefit of different diagnostic investigations. Fluoroscopy studies carry the greatest dose, but are very operator dependent, with variable degrees of radiation exposure. Although many barium investigations are being replaced by CT studies (e.g. enemas), fluoroscopy activity is increasing overall with the advancement of endovascular intervention techniques. CT is the 'workhorse' of a radiology department and carries significant radiation exposure risk. Although collimation and dose-reduction techniques are improving, if possible, always consider an alternative method of answering the diagnostic question. For example, if the patient is low risk, a lower dose ventilation/perfusion (V/Q) study may diagnose a pulmonary embolism rather than a CT chest.

 KEY POINTS

- Formal chest radiographs are acquired in a posterior–anterior (PA) orientation.
- The silhouette sign can accurately locate pathology to a particular lung lobe.
- Always consider radiation dose to the patient when requesting a radiological procedure.

History

A 45-year-old farm worker is bought to hospital by his wife. While changing the wheel of his tractor earlier today, the jack collapsed and the tyre landed on his left foot before roll-ing off. He felt an immediate sharp and stabbing pain which was exacerbated by walking. His foot began to swell despite ice and elevation. Worried that he may have fractured a bone they attended the minor injuries unit that evening.

He has no relevant past medical history but is a smoker of 20 pack-years.

Examination

Examination reveals a swollen left foot with bruising centred on the plantar arch. The patient is in continued discomfort, with the medial aspect of the foot being most tender over the first metatarsal. He is sent for a foot radiograph before further management is planned (Figure 87.1).

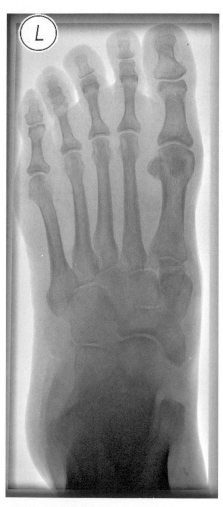

Questions
- What injury does this radiograph show?
- What joint and ligament is involved?
- Why is it important to recognize this injury?

Figure 87.1 Anterior–posterior (AP) radiograph of foot.

In a normal anterior–posterior (AP) radiograph of a foot, the medial aspect of the second metatarsal should align with the medial margin of the middle cuneiform. Figure 87.1 demonstrates an AP weight-bearing radiograph of the left foot. There is malalignment of the Lisfranc joint, with a homolateral 3 mm slip of the second to fifth metatarsals. No obvious fracture is seen and the remaining bones of the mid- and forefoot are intact and correctly located. These features are in keeping with a Lisfranc dislocation, and the patient should be referred to orthopaedics for further management.

The Lisfranc joint separates the bones of the midfoot, comprising the cuneiform and cuboid bones, from the metatarsals of the forefoot. Each cuneiform bone articulates with its first, second and third metatarsal, respectively, with the fourth and fifth metatarsals articulating with the cuboid bone. Stability of the joint is maintained by complex ligaments found on the plantar surface, which maintain alignment when weight-bearing. These ligaments are subject to significant shear forces on every step a person takes, and are put under increased pressure in athletes. The largest ligament is the Lisfranc ligament, which originates from the lateral aspect of the medial cuneiform bone, and inserts into the medial aspect of the second metatarsal. It is primarily responsible for stability of the whole joint, and maintains the plantar arch while preventing the second to fifth metatarsals slipping laterally when walking.

Following injury, the Lisfranc ligament may either be stretched (Lisfranc sprain) or completely torn. Joint stability and alignment is lost, causing diastasis between the first and second metatarsals and dislocation of the Lisfranc joint. Patients present acutely with soft tissue swelling, plantar bruising and pain on weight-bearing. Special attention should be given to those patients with sensory peripheral neuropathy (e.g. alcoholics and diabetics).

The injury is sustained either through longstanding repetitive strain placed upon the ligament (e.g. athletes), or from a direct axial load forcing the foot downwards while in rotation. The latter is often associated with bone fractures in combination with Lisfranc dislocation. When suspected, a patient should be referred for orthopaedic assessment with further imaging in the form of computed tomography (CT) to look for associated fractures (Figure 87.2), and magnetic resonance imaging (MRI) to assess ligament integrity. Without correction, normal biomechanics of the foot are lost, and the patient will develop irreversible osteoarthritic change with eventual incapacitating disability on a background of chronic pain.

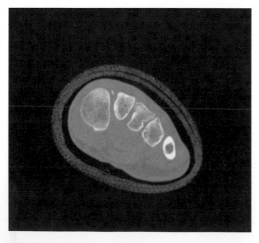

Figure 87.2 Unenhanced coronal CT image with bone windowing showing a bony fragment in between the first and second metatarsal bases indicative of a Lisfranc ligament rupture.

Treatment differs between institutions and is determined by joint stability. In a sprain where the Lisfranc ligament is intact, treatment is conservative with the foot immobilized in a cast for 6 weeks. When the joint is unstable, surgery is required with the insertion of screws and wires necessary to maintain reduction. The foot is immobilized in a cast, and the patient is non-weight-bearing for 3 months. The screws are eventually removed following satisfactory healing with clinical outcome dependent on restoration of normal alignment.

 KEY POINTS

- Bony misalignment can indicate ligamentous injury in the absence of bony injury.
- Two views of a bony joint, preferably at right angles to each other, should always be acquired.
- Patients should be referred for an MRI or CT scan if there is suspicion of bony/ligamentous injury.

History

A 37-year-old accountant has been referred to your outpatient clinic by his general practitioner (GP). He complains of vague abdominal discomfort, which is central, colicky and intermittent. He has been having these symptoms for as long as he can remember and was thought to have irritable bowel syndrome. They have recently been increasing in frequency and his new GP decided to investigate them further. There are no predisposing factors and he has tried several dietary changes with no resolution of symptoms. He denies any weight loss, change in bowel habit or vomiting, but suffered attacks on a weekly basis now. The pain subsides spontaneously after a few hours with no sequelae.

There is no relevant past medical history. He does not take any regular medication and denies allergy. He is a non-smoker, does regular exercise and lives with his wife and child.

Examination

Nothing abnormal was found on examination. A set of blood results taken last month are normal, and he has recently had a barium follow-through investigation (Figure 88.1).

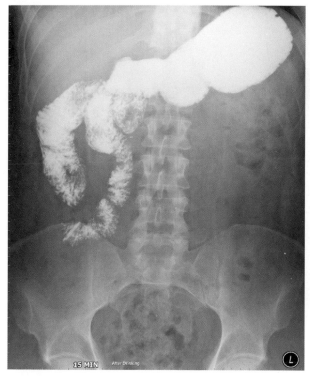

Figure 88.1 AP image from barium follow-through study.

Questions

- Describe the barium study.
- What is the abnormality demonstrated?
- What are the complications of this condition?

This is a single anterior–posterior (AP) image from a barium follow-through study, centred on the abdomen and pelvis. There is good contrast opacification of the stomach with normal distended appearances and no evidence of a filling defect. Barium is seen to pass freely into the duodenum and jejunum on this 15-minute film, with no evidence of stricture or obstruction. The pylorus and proximal duodenum are seen in the expected position, but the opacified distal duodenum fails to cross the midline, instead remaining on the right of the abdomen. The duodenal–jejunal (DJ) junction is abnormally located within the right upper quadrant, with opacified jejunum appearing to continue on the right side. Delayed images are required to see the position of the remaining small bowel and caecal pole.

Figure 88.2 shows an image from the same patient taken at 80 minutes following ingestion of barium and demonstrated continuation of the entire small bowel to the right of the midline. There is no evidence of stricture or obstruction. The caecal pole is located within the pelvis, but is medial to its expected position in the right iliac fossa. The hepatic flexure is abnormally positioned and lies within the left upper quadrant, with the entire large bowel seen to lie on the left side of the abdomen. These features indicate a diagnosis of malrotation.

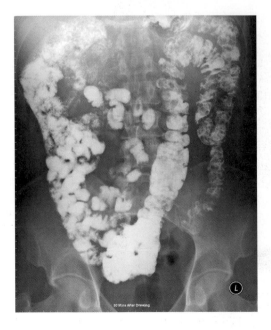

Figure 88.2 Subsequent image from barium follow-through.

During embryological development the primitive mid- and hindgut move out of the abdominal cavity and normally rotate 270 degrees anticlockwise on a mesentery around the central omphalomesenteric axis. This twisting movement allows the gut to pass under the primitive superior mesenteric vessels as they form, before re-entering the abdomen. The DJ flexure is then fixed to the base of the left hemidiaphragm by the ligament of Treitz, and the caecal pole is secured in the right lower quadrant.

If the primitive gut is secured to a mesentry that is shorter than usual, the gut cannot complete its full rotation, leaving the caecal pole and DJ junction in anatomically abnormal positions. This is termed 'malrotation', and is best diagnosed with a barium follow-through study, to identify the abnormal peritoneal fixation from the position of the bowel loops. On a CT scan, the position of the superior mesenteric vessels is reversed, with the superior mesenteric artery (SMA) positioned to the right of the superior mesenteric vein (SMV). Imaging studies demonstrate a variety of appearances depending on how much of the 270 degrees the bowel rotated before fixation, with a right-sided duodenum and jejunum being the commonest finding. Patients are often symptomatic as neonates and children, suffering from recurrent abdominal pain, distension and vomiting. Failure of the primitive gut to rotate at all results in the entire small bowel on the right side of the abdomen with the large bowel on the left, as in this case. These patients with non-rotation often present as adults, and describe a history of mild intermittent abdominal pain for as long as they can remember.

A short mesentry predisposes children to the complication of midgut volvulus. Most commonly presenting in the first 3 weeks of life, children present with bilious projectile vomiting and abdominal pain. This is a medial emergency and can lead to bowel infarction and death. Its characteristic features on a barium study demonstrate malrotation with a spiralling 'corkscrew' appearance to the bowel distal to the obstruction (Figure 88.3).

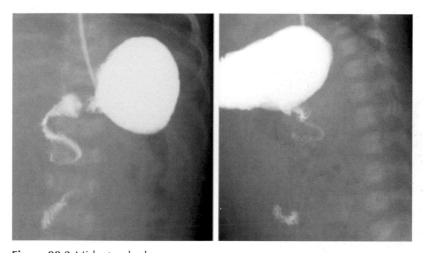

Figure 88.3 Midgut volvulus.

 KEY POINTS

- Oral contrast fluoroscopy studies have a high sensitivity for detecting malrotation.
- Normal embryological development involves a 270 degree anticlockwise rotation around a central omphalomesenteric axis.
- On CT scans, check the position of the SMA in relation to the SMV in cases of suspected malrotation.

History

A 57-year-old woman attends the hospital for a computed tomography (CT) scan. She was diagnosed with breast cancer 3 years previously and was successfully treated with a right mastectomy, radiotherapy and chemotherapy. Following breast reconstruction last year, a routine CT scan demonstrated no assessable disease and the patient was offered a clinic appointment for 6 months' time. Recently she has noticed some increasing pain the right upper quadrant of her abdomen and reported unexpected weight loss of over 2 kg. Informing her hospital consultant via telephone, the patient was asked to attend hospital for a blood test and repeat CT scan of the chest and abdomen. She is due to see the consultant in clinic tomorrow.

Examination

On the CT scan you find evidence of post-surgical change within the reconstructed right breast with no assessable disease above the diaphragm. Abdominal review demonstrates multiple areas of low attenuation within the liver, which are new compared to the previous CT, in keeping with hepatic metastases. Both kidneys are unobstructed and there is no evidence of portal vein thrombosis. To complete the report, you review the bony skeleton reconstructed in the sagittal plane for improved image interpretation (Figure 89.1).

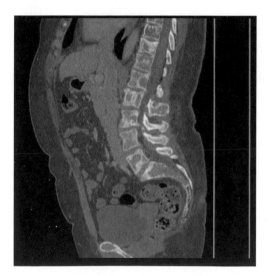

Figure 89.1 Sagittal reconstruction from a CT scan.

Questions

- What does the CT scan demonstrate?
- What are the common tumour types that cause this appearance?
- What further radiographic investigations should be considered?

This image is a sagittal reconstruction from a CT scan centred on the lower thoracic, lumbar and sacral spine. It has been windowed to improve bony resolution. It demonstrates multiple areas of well-defined reduced attenuation and loss of the normal bony architecture throughout the vertebral column and sacrum with evidence of posterior element involvement. They have a narrow zone of transition and are surrounded by areas of ill-defined sclerosis. The vertebral column retains a normal alignment and there is no loss of vertebral body height to suggest vertebral collapse. Within the limits of this single image, the cord appears capacious throughout, although review of the whole image series is recommended. The findings are in keeping with multilevel lytic bone metastases.

Secondary bone deposits are approximately 100 times more common than primary bone tumours.[1] Spread from the tumour haematogenously, via the lymphatics or through direct invasion, they have a predilection for parts of the skeleton with high marrow content, affecting the axial skeleton more often than the ribs and skull. Their presence alters the bone integrity, and patients are at increased risk of fracture despite normal physiological loads being applied, known as 'pathological fractures'. This is most marked in the spine, where vertebral compression fractures can cause spinal canal stenosis from retropulsed bone fragments, which can encroach on the spinal cord causing compression and neurological compromise. Spinal cord compression is a neurosurgical emergency.

Depending on cell type, tumour deposits upregulate either osteoclastic or osteoblastic activity, giving characteristic radiographic appearances. Those metastases with osteoclastic activity cause bone lysis, with soft tissue deposits destroying the adjacent bone and reducing the structural integrity. On X-ray, the bone can appear 'moth-eaten' and destroyed, with pain being the commonest clinical symptom. Osteoblastic metastases cause bone sclerosis, with new bone formation appearing as areas of increased density. The involved bones retain their normal morphology, but the heterotrophic bone has abnormal trabecular architecture, reducing the overall bone integrity. To confuse matters, some tumour types have metastases with both lytic and sclerotic components, and lytic bone metastases become sclerotic following treatment (e.g. radiotherapy or chemotherapy). A few metastases can also cause characteristic bone expansion and the common appearances are listed in Table 89.1.

Table 89.1 Common tumour appearances

Tumour type	Lytic	Sclerotic	Expansile
Lung	X		
Breast	X	X	
Prostate		X	
Kidney	X		X
Bowel	X		
Lymphoma	X	X	
Carcinoid		X	
Thyroid	X		X
Bladder		X	

Bone metastases are more likely to be multiple than solitary, and a combination of modalities such as plain X-ray, CT and MRI are used to assess bony metastatic disease. Bone scintigraphy, where radioactive phosphate particles are administered intravenously, is often appropriate in characterization of disease distribution and treatment response.

The whole body is imaged, and the normal physiological bone appearances are disturbed by areas of intense tracer uptake from sclerosis, or areas of photopenia from bone lysis. It is highly sensitive with relatively low radiation exposure, and is useful to localize areas of possible disease for further assessment.

Figure 89.2 shows a bone scintigraphy study from a patient with a prostate specific antigen (PSA) of >2000, with increased tracer uptake seen in the skull, both shoulders, shaft of both humeri and femora. There is also diffuse uptake of tracer noted in multiple ribs bilaterally as well as in multiple vertebrae at multiple levels. The proximal tibia, pelvis and right sterno-clavicular joints are also involved. Both kidneys are not visualized suggesting a 'superscan' consistent with extensive bone metastases from an underlying diagnosis of prostate cancer.

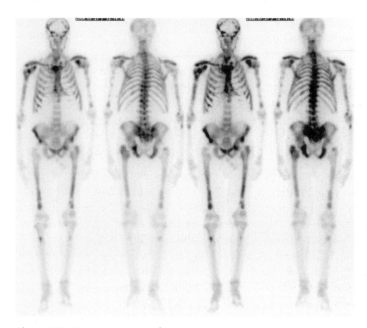

Figure 89.2 Bone scintigraphy images.

 KEY POINTS

- Bone metastases can be either lytic, sclerotic or mixed
- CT has a high sensitivity for resolving bony abnormality.
- Bone scintigraphy can be employed to assess the extent of bone involvement.

Reference

1. Dahnert, W. (2011) *Radiology Review Manual*, 7th edn. Philadelphia: Lippincott Williams and Wilkins.

History

A 48-year-old man has been referred by his general practitioner (GP) for further management. He complains of weight gain, tiredness and headache over the last few months with no resolution of symptoms despite diet and analgesia. Initially thought to be stress related, a screening blood test revealed normal biochemical markers other than a slightly low T4, low thyroid stimulating hormone (TSH) and low testosterone.

There is no relevant medical history. He is not taking regular medication and is a non-smoker. Living at home with his wife and children, he has taken several sick days recently because of his symptoms.

Examination

Examination reveals a tired looking Caucasian man in no obvious discomfort. His body mass index (BMI) is 26 (previously recorded at 23). He is afebrile, normotensive and with a regular pulse of 56 beats per minute. Cardiovascular, respiratory and abdominal examination is normal. On neurological examination, visual field assessment reveals a bitemporal hemianopia. A thyroid ultrasound scan and chest radiograph were normal, and a cranial computed tomography (CT) scan was arranged (Figures 90.1 and 90.2).

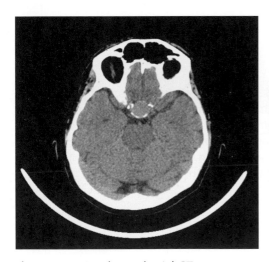

Figure 90.1 Unenhanced axial CT scan.

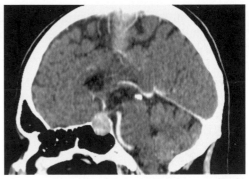

Figure 90.2 Enhanced sagittal CT scan.

Questions
- What does the CT scan show?
- Is there a differential for these appearances and what would you do next?
- What is the cause of the patient's symptoms and biochemical abnormality?

The two images of the same patient are taken from a cranial CT study before and after the infusion of intravenous contrast. The axial image (Figure 90.1) is unenhanced and acquired at the level of the cavernous sinus. The patient's head is slightly tilted to the right. Within the suprasellar space there is a soft tissue mass measuring approximately 20 × 17 mm which is well defined and isodense to the neighbouring brain tissue. It is of homogenous attenuation and displays curvilinear rim calcification. It is expanding the sellar turcica and splaying the cavernous sinus laterally. There is normal grey/white differentiation and no evidence of acute haemorrhage. The second image (Figure 90.2) is taken following the infusion of intravenous contrast and reformatted in the coronal plane. The soft tissue mass demonstrates avid uniform enhancement centred on the pituitary fossa with suprasellar extension towards the optic chiasm and third ventricle. The sella is expanded as before but there is no obvious breach of the sella floor or extension into the sphenoid sinus. Within the limits of these images, the basal cisterns are preserved throughout and there is no evidence of hydrocephalus or tentorial herniation.

The differential for a pituitary mass with suprasellar extension includes:

- pituitary adenoma;
- carotid artery aneurysm;
- meningioma;
- pituitary metastasis;
- pituitary lymphoma;
- pituitary abscess;
- Rathke's cleft cyst.

From this differential list, pituitary abscess and Rathke's cleft cyst can be discounted as the pituitary mass is of homogeneous soft tissue density and the patient is not clinically septic or unwell. Pituitary metastasis and lymphoma are very rare and would be an unlikely diagnosis considering there are no other systemic symptoms. The patient should undergo magnetic resonance imaging (MRI) to characterize the mass further, with neurology/neurosurgery referral for outpatient follow-up (Figure 90.3).

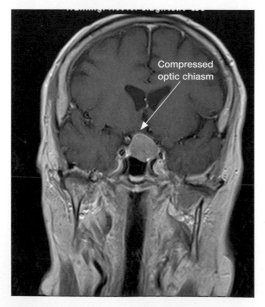

Figure 90.3 T1-weighted gadolinium-enhanced coronal MRI image demonstrating an enhancing pituitary mass lesion with suprasellar extension. The arrow highlights the compression of the optic chiasm. This requires urgent surgical attention so as to preserve vision.

This patient has a pituitary adenoma, which is a slow growing tumour of the anterior pituitary gland. Despite being benign, patients are frequently symptomatic depending on its size and functioning status. Pituitary adenomas are classified into macro- or microadenomas. Patients with pituitary microadenomas (<10 mm) often present with symptoms of hormonal imbalance resulting from functionally active tumours, most commonly prolactin secreting with symptoms of amenorrhoea and infertility; instability of the adrenocortical, somatostatin and gonadotrophin axis can also occur.

In this case, the patient has a pituitary macroadenoma (>10 mm) with symptoms resulting from mass effect related to tumour bulk. Compression of normal pituitary tissue by tumour has resulted in loss of TSH secretion and a clinically hypothyroid patient. In addition, suprasellar tumour extension is causing compression of the optic chiasm and stretching of the prechiasmic optic nerve. This is highlighted on the MRI study and is the cause of the bitemporal hemianopia. With no intervention, the tumour will continue to grow and he will be at risk of visual loss, obstructive hydrocephalus and carotid artery involvement. This patient was referred to neurosurgery with successful tumour removal and complete symptom resolution.

 KEY POINTS

- The suprasellar space should be a review area when viewing unenhanced CT images.
- The use of intravenous contrast improves diagnostic interpretation.
- Always looks for optic chiasm compression in suprasellar masses.

History

A 71-year-old man is referred to the vascular surgical team with right leg pain. He is known to suffer from atherosclerotic peripheral vascular disease and is currently being treated conservatively for claudication. The pain in his right leg started suddenly 3 hours previously, with an achy discomfort that is not relieved by simple analgesia or positioning. Limited by pain, his mobility has reduced to only a few steps, and he reports increasing discoloration of his right foot compared to the left.

His relevant medical history includes type 2 diabetes mellitus, hypertension and angina. He is an ex-smoker of 40 pack-years. His drug history includes aspirin, metformin, isosorbide mononitrate and a calcium channel blocker. He takes sublingual glyceryl trinitrate as required.

Examination

Having been treated by the accident and emergency department for his pain, examination reveals a mottled right foot and reduced popliteal and pedal pulses compared to the left side. Femoral pulses are symmetrical and strong bilaterally, with no evidence of an expansile pulsatile abdominal mass. A computed tomography (CT) angiogram is performed which suggests a right common femoral stenosis, and the interventional radiologists are approached for advice (Figure 91.1).

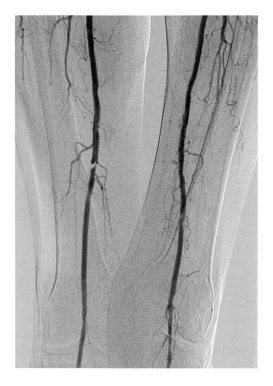

Figure 91.1 Lower limb angiogram.

Questions

- What type of study is this and what does it show?
- What treatment options are available in this case?
- What factors need to be considered when using radiographic contrast agents?

Figure 91.1 is a single view acquired during an angiogram of the lower limbs. It is a procedure performed by the interventional radiologists on a fluoroscopy table, with the patient in the supine position. With a sterile technique, a needle is passed into the common femoral artery (CFA) under ultrasound guidance and subcutaneous local anaesthetic cover. In this case, a retrograde puncture of the left side was made to image the arteries of both legs, however an antegrade puncture technique is sometimes preferable in certain situations. Adopting the Seldinger technique, a guidewire is passed via the puncture needle into the aorta, and this is used to railroad a sheath and 'pigtail' multihole catheter. Positioning the catheter at the aortic bifurcation, 15 mL of contrast is pumped at 8 mL/s with digital subtraction images acquired of the opacified lower limb arteries.

A short tight stenosis of the mid superficial femoral artery on the right side is demonstrated, with the artery narrowed by approximately 80 per cent by a flow-limiting atherosclerotic plaque. There is a paucity of collateral vessels suggesting an acute obstruction. There is good run-off of the distal vessels. Both superficial femoral arteries demonstrate a background of mild atherosclerotic calcification.

Although surgery in the form of endarterectomy or bypass could relieve this stenosis, an open operation would carry significant risk and leave the patient with a visible scar. An endovascular repair through the left CFA puncture is preferable, leaving the patient with only a small pinhole scar in the groin and conserving the tissues of the right leg.

Crossing the aortic bifurcation, the stenosis can be transgressed with an atraumatic hydrophilic guidewire. This can then guide the passage of a balloon-mounted bare metal stent to the level of the stenosis. Balloon inflation (Figure 91.2) compresses the atherosclerotic plaque and delivers the stent to exert radial force and maintain continued patency long term (Figure 91.3).

The post-procedure angiogram (Figure 91.4) reveals a good response to treatment with improved blood flow to aid symptomatic relief. The sheath and catheter are removed and haemostasis of the groin achieved by manual compression. The patient will require dual antiplatelet therapy to aid stent patency.

Radiographic contrast media is used in all aspects of radiology to enhance tissue contrast and improve diagnostic interpretation. Barium, water and air can all be used in certain examinations (e.g. barium enema) but this is not suitable for intravenous usage in CT and angiographic studies. Iodine, with its high atomic number, has strong photoelectric X-ray absorption characteristics that make it ideal for use in intravenous contrast media. Injecting a predefined volume and imaging at a specific time allows for tissue enhancement characteristics to be determined and improves the contrast between soft tissues (Figure 91.4).

Before referring a patient for a study that involves the use of iodinated contrast, certain parameters need to be checked. There are documented allergies to contrast media, and also potential crossover in sensitive atopic individuals with shellfish and certain fruits (e.g. strawberries). Contrast media is predominantly renally excreted and patients require a degree of endogenous renal function to clear the injected contrast load. Intravenous contrast is also nephrotoxic and can precipitate renal failure in predisposed patients. It is important, therefore, to check a patient's renal function prior to imaging to alleviate this potential risk. Adequate hydration before and after the use of intravenous contrast media is also recommended.

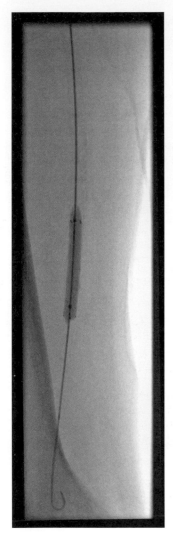

Figure 91.2

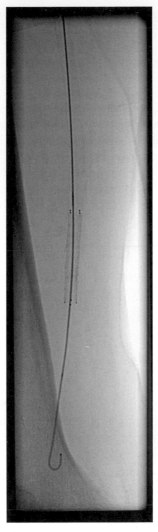

Figure 91.3

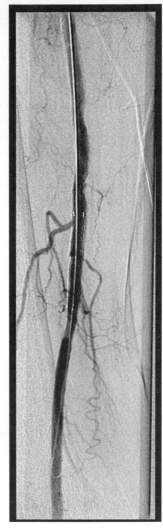

Figure 91.4 Post-procedure angiogram.

 KEY POINTS

- Always review all imaging available before proceeding with an interventional procedure.
- Stent insertion is avoided if possible at areas of flexion to avoid stent kinking.
- Always check a patient's renal function before initiating the use of intravenous contrast.

History

Following her second year of foundation training, a 26-year-old junior doctor has decided to spend a year in Australia gaining further experience. Having successfully gained sponsorship by the Northern Sydney Central Coast Health Authority, she has to be certified medically fit by a recognized senior physician to comply with immigration policy. This involves completing a medical questionnaire, satisfying a medical examination, completing a series of screening blood tests and having a normal chest radiograph with no evidence of communicable disease.

She feels well and has no relevant past medical history. Other than being an occasional smoker there is no significant findings at history or physical examination.

Examination

Her blood results are as follows: white cell count (WCC) 9.4×10^9/L, Na 137 mmol/L, bilirubin 9 µmol/L, haemoglobin 11.6 g/dL, K 4.2 mmol/L, alanine aminotransferase (ALT) 27 IU/L, mean corpuscular volume (MCV) 78 fL, urea 4.1 mmol/L, alkaline phosphatase 146 IU/L, HIV negative, creatinine 87 µmol/L, albumin 41 g/L. Chest radiograph is shown in Figure 92.1.

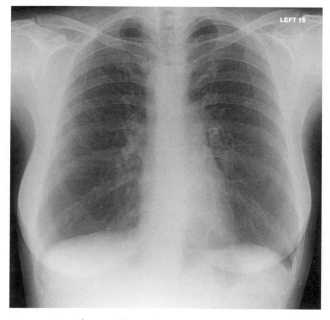

Figure 92.1 Chest radiograph.

Questions

- What normal variant is found on this chest radiograph?

ANSWER 92

Figure 92.1 is a chest radiograph of an adult female patient. It is not rotated and there is adequate penetration with optimal inspiratory effort made. The heart is of normal orientation and size (cardiothoracic ratio 30/12 cm), with both hilar correctly positioned with normal appearances. Cardiomediastinal assessment demonstrates a right-sided aortic arch. The lungs are clear and free from active disease. There is no evidence of old *Mycobacterium tuberculosis* exposure. Bone review is normal. There is no pneumothorax or evidence of free air under the diaphragm.

Normal aortic anatomy: The aorta is divided into the ascending thoracic aorta, arch of the aorta, descending thoracic aorta and abdominal aorta. The ascending aorta begins at the aortic root running superiorly and anteriorly, adjacent to the right side of the sternum. It is enclosed with the pulmonary trunk in a sheath of serous pericardium and is in continuation with the arch of the aorta. Lying behind the manubrium of the sternum, the aortic arch runs superiorly, posteriorly and from left to right anterior to the trachea. The arch gives rise to the brachiocephalic artery, left carotid artery and left subclavian artery as it runs across the mediastinum to become the descending thoracic aorta. This descends inferiorly as a posterior mediastinal structure, piercing the diaphragm at the level of the twelfth thoracic vertebra and is in continuity with the abdominal aorta.

A right aortic arch is an embryological variant with persistence of the right arch and right descending aorta while undergoing regression of the left side. Seen in approximately 2 per cent of the western population, its course within the chest is to the right of the trachea and oesophagus, crossing the midline in the lower thorax to pierce the diaphragm in the anatomically correct position. Its incidence increases in congenital heart disease (e.g. tetralogy of Fallot), and is commonly associated with one of three aberrant vascular anomalies:

- **Right aortic arch with aberrant left subclavian artery**: This is the commonest right aortic arch anomaly and is associated with cardiac septal defects and coarctation. The patient is usually asymptomatic but its positioning predisposes to aortic torsion in adulthood. The left carotid artery is the first branch of the aortic arch with an aberrant left subclavian artery arising from the proximal descending aorta.
- **Right aortic arch with mirror image branching**: As the second commonest right aortic arch anomaly, this is caused by embryological interruption of the arch between the left subclavian artery and the descending aorta, most commonly just distal to the ductus arteriosus. The great vessels branch opposite to the anatomicial norm, and patients are often symptomatic, being strongly associated with cyanotic heart disease (e.g. truncus arteriosus).
- **Right aortic arch with isolated left subclavian artery**: In this third most common scenario, the aortic arch is interrupted between the left common carotid artery and the left subclavian artery. The result is a left subclavian artery arising from the left pulmonary artery, and the patient is symptomatic with congenital subclavian steal syndrome.

A right aortic arch is a normal anatomical variant. Having survived into adulthood with no symptoms, it is highly unlikely that this incidental finding is of any clinical consequence. The student was passed fit to travel, and had a successful year in Australia.

 KEY POINTS

- The normal aortic arch runs superiorly, posteriorly and from left to right anterior to the trachea.
- A right-sided aortic arch is seen in 2 per cent of the population.
- There are often concomitant aberrant vascular anomalies with a right-sided aortic arch.

History

An intravenous urogram (IVU) study is requested on a 41-year-old man who has presented with right flank pain. His symptoms started 3 days ago with a dull pain on his right side just below his ribs, which has remained constant and is not relieved by simple analgesia. He attended his local accident and emergency department last night as the pain woke him from sleep, and a presumptive diagnosis of a right-sided renal stone was made. He was placed on appropriate analgesia.

He had no relevant medical history until last year when he experienced an acute but short-lived pain on his left side while on holiday in Africa. Returning to the United Kingdom, his general practitioner (GP) retrospectively diagnosed a renal stone and investigations showed a slightly elevated serum calcium and parathyroid hormone level. He is currently being investigated for hypercalcaemia and further nuclear medicine studies are scheduled next month.

Examination

His results today demonstrate a deterioration in renal function (creatinine 320 μmol/L) compared to a normal baseline last month. His urine dipstick is positive for microscopic blood but free from white cells and protein. On examination he is more comfortable following analgesia, but there is a pain on deep palpation and a fullness to the right side of his abdomen compared to the left. The intravenous urograms are shown in Figure 93.1.

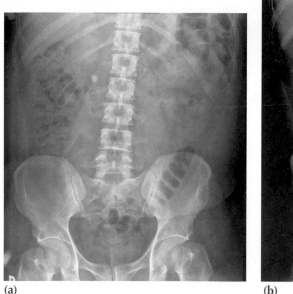

(a)

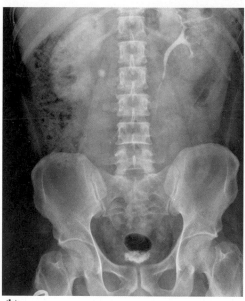

(b)

Figure 93.1 Intravenous urograms: (a) control; (b) 20 minutes post contrast.

Questions

- What does this IVU study demonstrate?
- What imaging modalities are available to characterize this type of problem?
- How should this patient be treated?

These are two images from an IVU study. The control film (Figure 93.1a) demonstrates a solitary well-defined calcified focus measuring 12 mm overlying the right pelvico-ureteric junction (PUJ)/upper ureter. There is no other radio-opacity overlying the renal tracts and both kidneys appear of equal size and shape. Post intravenous contrast administration (Figure 93.1b) there is asymmetrical excretion of contrast, with normal appearances to the left kidney and ureter, but delayed excretion and a persistent nephrogram on the right. No contrast is seen within the right collecting system on the post-micturition 20-minute film, suggesting a partially obstructed right renal system.

On delayed imaging at 4 hours (Figure 93.2), there is excretion of contrast into a dilated pelvicocalyceal system, with the distal pelvis measuring approximately 11 mm. There is a faint trace of contrast seen within the right mid ureter, with additional contrast collecting in the bladder compared to the 20-minute post-micturition film. These findings are in keeping with a partially obstructed right renal system, most likely caused by a renal stone at the PUJ/proximal ureter.

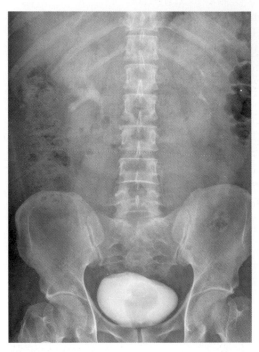

Figure 93.2 Delayed imaging at 4 hours.

Nephrolithiasis is the most common cause of renal calcification with over 10 per cent of the western population developing a stone by the age of 70 years.[1] The majority of renal stones (80 per cent) are made of calcium oxalate/calcium phosphate and are commonly associated with primary and secondary hypercalcaemia. The remaining renal stones have a mineral composition of either cystine or magnesium ammonium phosphate (struvite). Rarely, renal stones can be formed from either uric acid, xanthine or a mucopolysaccaride matrix, and it is important to remember this, as these stones are radiolucent and therefore radiologically invisible.

Other than an IVU, other imaging modalities include:

- **Ultrasound**: The renal stone is highly echogenic against the grey renal parenchyma, with an acoustic shadow often projected deep to the stone. Ultrasound also carries a high sensitivity of detecting pelvicocalyceal dilatation and does not expose the patient to ionizing radiation. Its limiting factor is operator dependence. Small, non-obstructing stones may be poorly visualized due to renal pelvis fat, which is also echogenic.
- **Computed tomography (CT)**: Non-contrast CT-KUB (kidneys, ureter, bladder) is the gold standard and is highly sensitive for renal stone detection and characterization. The radiation dose is low and exam time is short (less than 5 minutes), with no risk of nephropathy as intravenous contrast is not required. Stone size, position and density can be assessed to guide treatment (e.g. lithotripsy or percutaneous nephrolithotomy (PCNL)). CT-KUB is replacing IVU as the preferred imaging modality for renal stone disease.
- **Nuclear medicine**: There is a limited role for both MAG3 and DTPA (diethylene triamine pentaacetic acid) studies in cases of nephrolithiasis, with the stone appearing as an area of photopenia on a background of homogeneous uptake. In an obstructed system the studies are more useful and can demonstrate renal perfusion abnormalities and can be used to compare the split function of both kidneys.
- **Magnetic resonance imaging (MRI)**: This modality has no significant role in the diagnosis of renal stone disease but may do in the future.

In this patient, an obstructed right renal system and deteriorating renal function needs to have definitive treatment to decompress the renal pelvis and preserve right kidney function. Options include a percutaneous nephrostomy inserted under fluoroscopy guidance by the interventional radiologists (see Case 71). However, the nephrostomy drainage catheter can only remain in place for a limited time and this procedure carries risks of infection and bleeding. The preferred alternative is a ureteric stent which can be placed in a retrograde fashion during cystoscopy over a guidewire. The 'double-J' stents have multiple perforations and can bypass the stone, allowing pelvicocalyceal decompression. The ureteric stent can remain in place for up to 3 months while a definitive decision on stone removal is made, and is then easily removed during a repeat cystoscopy procedure when necessary (Figure 93.3).

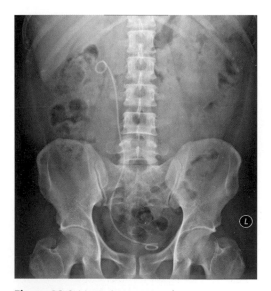

Figure 93.3 Ureteric stent in place.

KEY POINTS

- The majority of renal stones are radio-opaque and are made of calcium oxalate/phosphate.
- Non-contrast CT (CT-KUB) is the gold standard investigation for characterizing renal stone disease.
- Obstructed and infected collecting systems require urgent decompression, usually via nephrostomy insertion.

Reference

1. Dahnert, W. (2007) *Radiology Review Manual*, 6th edn. Philadelphia: Lippincott Williams and Wilkins.

History

A 42-year-old woman is bought to the accident and emergency department by her husband complaining of headache. Her symptoms started a few hours earlier with the sudden onset of sharp stabbing pain at the back of her head. This rapidly progressed and soon became the worst headache she had ever had. Despite simple analgesia and rest, the headache did not subside and the pain caused her to vomit several times. There has been no altered consciousness but her husband was concerned by her restlessness and agitation, and brought her to hospital.

The patient has a past medical history of asthma, which is well controlled on inhalers provided by her general practitioner (GP). She also has annual review with the hospital nephrologists for a history of polycystic kidney disease.

Examination

She is irritable and looks unwell. She is hypertensive (170/110) and has a regular pulse of 105 beats per minute. There is neck stiffness, and worsening of her headache on straight leg raising but no focal neurology. Ophthalmoscopy is not tolerated and the patient asks you to turn the lights off as they are hurting her eyes. A computed tomography (CT) scan was performed (Figure 94.1).

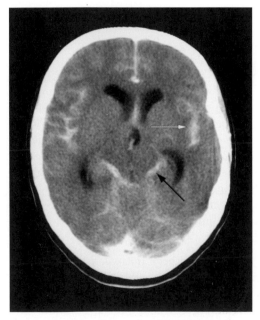

Figure 94.1 Unenhanced axial CT scan.

Questions

- What does the CT scan demonstrate?
- Why was this patient at increased risk?
- What would you do if the CT scan had been normal?

This image is a single slice from an unenhanced CT scan taken at the level of the basal ganglia. There is widespread abnormal high attenuation with a gyriform distribution within both cerebral hemispheres. This high attenuation material is denser than adjacent brain parenchyma but less dense than bone and represents acute blood. In the image, arrows demonstrate acute blood replacing CSF within the Sylvian fissure (white arrow) and quadrigeminal cistern (black arrow). There is mass effect with sulcal effacement and the lateral/third ventricles are prominent in keeping with hydrocephalus. Some acute blood is seen within the third ventricle at the expected origin of the aqueduct of Sylvius. This patient has therefore suffered an acute subarachnoid haemorrhage (SAH) with hydrocephalus.

Subarachnoid haemorrhage is defined as blood collected between the pia and arachnoid mater. Clinically, patients with an SAH commonly present with an acute severe occipital headache ('thunderclap') with associated vomiting, altered conscious state and agitation. Unenhanced cranial CT demonstrates acute blood (white – HU 60–70) within the cerebro-spinal fluid (CSF) spaces. Large haemorrhages can be easily seen, but smaller bleeds can be more difficult.

Causes of SAH include:

- ruptured aneurysm,
- AV malformation,
- hypertensive haemorrhage,
- haemorrhage from tumour,
- intracranial infection,
- blood dyscrasias, and
- anticoagulation.

Adult polycystic kidney disease (APKD) is an autosomal dominant genetic condition, which is slow to progress but has 100 per cent penetration in the affected individual. Multiple thin-walled cysts form within native kidneys. Commonly causing pain, haematuria and proteinuria, unrestricted cyst growth replaces normal renal parenchyma, eventually causing renal failure. The patient is also at increased risk of developing renal cell carcinoma. APKD has associations with cysts in other organs (e.g. liver and pancreas), mitral valve prolapse and saccular 'berry' aneurysms of the cerebral arteries (3–13 per cent).[1] These aneurysms tend to be multifocal and rupture of any aneurysm causes blood to leak into the subarachnoid space and SAH.

If the CT scan in a patient with this suspicious history had been normal, a lumbar puncture would need to be considered as a normal cranial CT does not exclude small SAH (sensitivity 90 per cent).[1] Lumbar puncture is essential to confirm the presence of normal or altered blood (xanthochromia) within the circulating CSF that bathes the brain. Any blood in the CSF space can cause obstruction and put the patient at risk of communicating/non-communicating hydrocephalus and death. Clinicians often feel reassured by requesting a cranial CT to exclude the absolute contraindication of raised intracranial pressure (ICP) before lumbar puncture to reduce the risk of 'coning.' However, cranial CT is not a sensitive exclusion modality,[2] and full clinical assessment looking for the stigmata of raised ICP would be advised.

KEY POINTS

- In an SAH, blood collects between the pia and arachnoid mater.
- An unenhanced CT scan needs to be performed in any patient suspected of having a SAH.
- A normal CT scan does not exclude a small SAH or raised intracranial pressure.

References

1. Dahnert, W. (2007) *Radiology Review Manual*, 6th edn. Philadelphia: Lippincott Williams and Wilkins.
2. Winkler, F., Kastenbauer, S., Yousry, T.A. *et al.* (2002) Discrepancies between brain CT imaging and severely raised intracranial pressure proven ventriculostomy in adults with pneumococcal meningitis. *Journal of Neurology* 249: 1292–97.

History

You are asked to see a 32-year-old Afro-Caribbean man who complains of feeling generally unwell for the last week. He has had a low-grade fever that has not resolved despite bed rest and anti-pyrexial medication. He denies having a cough or any urinary symptoms and is usually a fit and active person. Over the last 2 days he has noticed a red rash on his legs that is becoming increasingly hot and tender, and also complains of facial swelling with an achy discomfort in his jaw. He has also had to stop wearing his contact lenses as his eyes have become red and irritable.

Examination

On examination he looks tired with red conjunctiva and a temperature of 38.1°C. There is smooth swelling of the parotids bilaterally with tenderness on palpation. His cardiovascular, respiratory and abdominal examination is normal but there is an ill-defined rash on the anterior aspect of both his shins that is raised, nodular and tender.

A full septic screen is performed and while the blood results are awaited, a chest radiograph is performed (Figure 95.1).

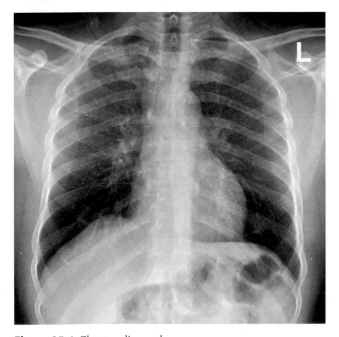

Figure 95.1 Chest radiograph.

Questions

- What does the chest radiograph demonstrate?
- How could a diagnosis be confirmed?
- What are the extrathoracic manifestations of this disease?

This is a posterior–anterior (PA) chest radiograph of an adult male patient, which has adequate inspiration, penetration and is not rotated. There is bilateral hilar enlargement with widening of the paratracheal stripe and loss of the normal convexity to the aortopulmonary window. These features are in keeping with lymph node enlargement and suggest the '1-2-3 sign' of Garland's triad. The lung parenchyma also demonstrates pathology, with reticular nodular shadowing bilaterally in a mid and upper zone distribution with basal sparing. The nodules are small (<2 mm) and there is no evidence of cavitation, pneumothorax or pleural effusion. The heart is of normal size and bone review is unremarkable.

Taking account of the ethnicity, history and examination of this patient, the top differential for these appearances would be acute sarcoidosis (Lofgren's syndrome). In the absence of an infective cause, biochemical and radiological findings are helpful, although definitive diagnosis relies on obtaining tissue by procedures such as transbronchial biopsy at bronchoscopy. The following should be noted:

- serum levels of angiotensin-converting enzyme (ACE) can be elevated in normal individuals;
- on chest radiograph, as well as the typical features described above, a more chronic picture can demonstrate parenchmyal volume loss and fibrosis, pleural effusions and mediastinal/hilar 'egg-shell' calcification;
- high-resolution computed tomography (HRCT) may be useful (Figure 95.2).

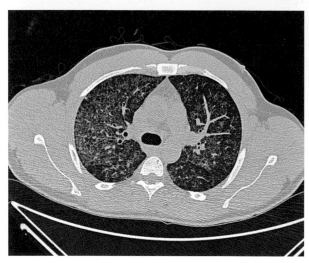

Figure 95.2 HRCT scan.

Although bilateral hilar adenopathy is the hallmark of this disease, the lung parenchyma is involved in approximately two-thirds of cases. High-resolution (thin, 1 mm) slices confirm reticular shadowing related to thickening of the interlobular septae from the interstitial lung disease. However, the presence and distribution of additional nodules is key to the diagnosis. The nodules can vary in size (2–4cm) and are caused by lymphoid hyperplasia related to the granulomatous response. Histologically, therefore, the nodules have a peri-lymphatic distribution and follow the course of the arterioles and bronchioles and are termed 'bronchovascular' in distribution. The nodules are most conspicuous along the thickened lung fissures, and give a 'beaded' appearance, which is demonstrated in Figure 95.2 particularly along the oblique fissure of the left lung. HRCT features in chronic disease can demonstrate fibrosis and loss of lung volume causing dilatation of the distal airways. This is termed 'traction bronchiectasis'.

Sarcoidosis is a multisystem granulomatous disease of unknown aetiology, and although thoracic manifestation is the commonest presentation, other organs are affected as follows:

- **Skin**: Cutaneous plaques, nodules and scarring can occur and are collectively termed 'lupus pernio'. More acutely, the patient can suffer from erythema nodosum where the skin is red and hot with tender nodularity.
- **Gastrointestinal**: Plaques and nodular granulomas can cause mucosal fold thickening anywhere along the gastrointestinal tract. This is most commonly seen in the stomach, followed by the colon, oesophagus and small bowel. Chronic involvement results in stricture formation with luminal narrowing.
- **Hepatobiliary**: Upper abdominal viscera involvement primarily causes organomegally. Late in the disease, granuloma formation can cause hepatic nodularity, however the patients often remain asymptomatic.
- **Bone**: Osseous involvement is a radiologist's favourite, most commonly affecting the hands and feet. Granuloma formation within the bone medulla causes loss of normal trabeculation resulting in a characteristic reticular 'lace-like' appearance. The overlying cortex demonstrates periosteal reaction and subperiosteal resorption mimicking hyperparathyroid disease.
- **Neurological**: Although a rare entity of the disease, cranial nerve palsies are the commonest manifestation (e.g. bilateral VIIth) with cerebral granuloma formation infrequently presenting as a space-occupying lesion.

KEY POINTS

- The presence of Garland's triad on a chest radiograph is highly suggestive of thoracic sarcoidosis.
- Lung nodules demonstrate a bronchovascular distribution on HRCT.
- As a multisystem granulomatous disease, sarcoidosis can affect any organ in the body.

History

A 58-year-old woman with a history of lung cancer has had a chest drain inserted for resolution of a unilateral right-sided pleural effusion. Since its insertion, the patient has noticed that the skin at the insertion site is continuing to slowly swell. This is exacerbated on coughing. She denies any shortness of breath or pain, and there is no evidence of active haemorrhage.

Examination

Examination reveals an ill-defined fullness to the right lateral chest wall, which has increased in size over the last few days. It is soft and compressible with nodularity felt on light palpation. The clinicians are concerned about basal crepitations over the area on auscultation with no evidence of a vascular bruit. The patient's blood results are unchanged from admission and a chest radiograph has been taken to assess positioning of the chest drain (Figure 96.1).

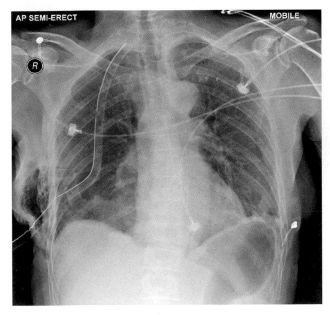

Figure 96.1 Chest radiograph.

Questions
- What does this chest radiograph demonstrate?
- What are the common causes of this finding?
- How should the patient be treated for this condition?

ANSWER 96

Figure 96.1 is an anterior–posterior (AP) semi-erect chest radiograph of an adult female patient. It is adequately penetrated with slight rotation. There is an intercostal chest drain within the right hemithorax with its tip positioned at the right apex. There is a small right-sided pleural effusion but no evidence of pneumothorax. The lungs are clear of any consolidation or collapse and the cardiomediastinal boarders are within normal limits. The soft tissues of the right lateral chest wall are expanded at the site of the chest drain insertion with locules of low-density gas projected within a subcutaneous distribution. These are confined to the right side with no cranial extension. These features are consistent with surgical emphysema of the right chest wall.

Surgical emphysema (also referred to as subcutaneous emphysema) occurs when gas collects within the subcutaneous tissues. It is able to track freely along the fascial planes, separating the tissue layers and causing distension. This is an enormous potential space and gas follows the path of least resistance limited only by the integrity of the overlying skin. Without correction of the underlying insult, the patient can become very swollen in appearance (Figure 96.2), with clinical examination revealing a unique 'crackling' sound akin to having crumpled tissue paper under the skin. Separation of the tissue planes is painless, with mild discomfort caused by increased skin tension and their bloated appearance.

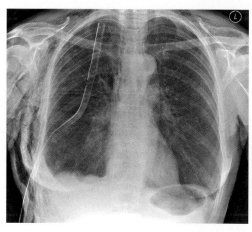

Figure 96.2 Chest radiograph showing swollen appearance.

Causes include:

- Infection: In susceptible patients (e.g. people with diabetes) the presence of a gas-forming organism under the skin will produce subcutaneous emphysema. When associated with tissue death, this gas gangrene requires surgical debridement to clear the organism, most commonly *Clostridium perfringens*.
- Trauma: Any form of blunt or penetrating trauma that disrupts the parietal covering of an air-containing organ (e.g. lung or intestinal tract) will form a conduit for air to move into the subcutaneous tissues along a favourable pressure gradient. This is most commonly seen in pneumothoraces associated with rib fractures or stabbings where a shard of bone or the knife pierces the parietal pleura. During expiration, air is forced into the subcutaneous space. Similarly, Boerhaave's syndrome with a ruptured

oesophagus will cause a pneumomediastinum and air can track into the subcutaneous tissues of the neck.

- **Spontaneous:** Patients with chronic lung disease (e.g. asthma, chronic obstructive pulmonary disease (COPD), cystic fibrosis) can suffer a spontaneous pneumothorax. If associated with disruption of the visceral pleura, air will track via the mediastinum to the subcutaneous space. This is also seen in intubated patients with barotraumas from ventilation pressures.
- **Iatrogenic:** The commonest cause of subcutaneous emphysema is following medical intervention or surgery. In the case described, the chest drain inserted for drainage of a pleural effusion has formed a conduit with the subcutaneous space. Air from a subclinical pneumothorax is leaking around the drain at the intercostal space and accumulating in the adjacent tissue. This drain is appropriately sited, however a fenestrated chest drain that is incorrectly placed with some of the drain holes outside the chest cavity will also cause subcutaneous emphysema. This is an important review area when reporting chest radiographs following drain insertion.

Having removed the original insult, the treatment for surgical emphysema is conservative. Air within the subcutaneous tissues will be slowly reabsorbed over a few weeks with no repercussions, but correction of the causative agent (e.g. pneumothorax) is essential to prevent reaccumulation.

 KEY POINTS

- Surgical emphysema occurs when gas accumulates within the subcutaneous tissues.
- Tracking along fascial planes, patients can become enormously distended and uncomfortable.
- When placing a fenestrated chest drain, ensure all drain holes lie within the chest cavity to avoid surgical emphysema.

History

You are asked by a junior doctor to review the chest radiograph of an 80-year-old man electively admitted for a pacemaker box change. Previously treated at another institution, there are no radiographs available for comparison. The patient is medically well and does not give a history of recent trauma. His past medical history includes previous syncope related to heart block, and he recalls a series of operations in his 20s for the treatment of tuberculosis.

Examination

On examination the patient is comfortable at rest with normal observations. Inspection reveals a right chest wall deformity and signs consistent with previous surgery. There is reduced lung expansion on the right, with reduced air entry at the apex and an area that is dull to percussion compared to the contralateral side. A chest radiograph is performed as part of the admission process (Figure 97.1).

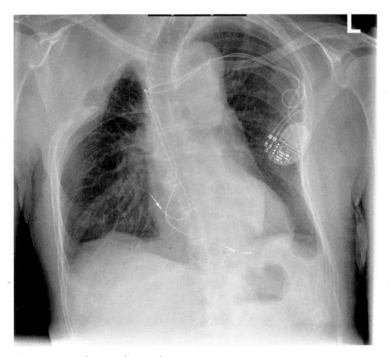

Figure 97.1 Chest radiograph.

Questions

- What does the chest radiograph demonstrate?
- What is this procedure and why was it performed?
- What other methods of treating this disease were employed before drug therapy?

ANSWER 97

Figure 97.1 is a frontal chest radiograph of an adult male patient, which is of adequate penetration but is rotated to the left. There is thoracic asymmetry, with a right-sided chest wall deformity centred on the upper zone. There has been surgical removal of the first five ribs on the right and corresponding transverse processes of the spine, with normal appearances of the ipsilateral clavicle and scapula. The right lung apex demonstrates volume loss from medialization and compression of the adjacent chest wall. There is no pleural effusion or pneumothorax and the changes appear chronic. Of note, there is a dual wire cardiac pacing device and the left hemithorax has normal appearances. These findings are characteristic of previous thoracoplasty for the treatment of pulmonary tuberculosis.

Mycobacterium tuberculosis was first described by Robert Koch in 1882. As an aerobic bacteria, it has an affinity for the lung apices where there is a higher ventilation perfusion ratio. The treatment for tuberculosis has radically changed over the last 100 years to the current 6-month regime starting with four drugs. Before the introduction of drug therapy, several methods of 'collapse therapy' existed, all with the common aim of reducing ventilation in the affected area. Thoracoplasty was practised until the 1960s, and an estimated 30 000 procedures were performed in the UK between 1951 and 1960.[1] Clinicians should be aware of the characteristic chest appearances, as it is still practised today in developing countries where the cost of chemotherapy is deemed excessive, and has been proposed in extensively resistant disease. In India, 139 thoracoplasties were performed between 1992 and 1997.[2] Cor pulmonale may result from the restrictive lung defect, particularly if the residual lung is affected by chronic obstructive pulmonary disease (COPD).

Thoracoplasty is commonly a three-stage procedure, with the 'modern' technique, as described in 1949, involving the eventual removal of the first to seventh ribs with their transverse processes and the angle of the scapula.[3] The superior lateral chest wall is then compressed towards the mediastinum, collapsing the affected upper lobe. Dewan *et al.* document a 66 per cent success rate in modern-day practice.[2]

Although thoracoplasty was widely used, other causes of 'collapse therapy' include the following:

- **Pneumothorax:** Forcibly introducing air into the pleural cavity, causing iatrogenic collapse of the lung, was deemed in 1820 a 'ray of sunshine in the dark history of tuberculosis'.[4] As the air was reabsorbed, frequent repeat procedures were necessary. Pneumoperitoneum was used for disease at the lung bases.
- **Internal pneumolysis:** Visceral/parietal adhesions were internally cauterized under direct vision with a thoracoscope before forcible pneumothorax collapse.
- **Oleothorax:** It was thought that the use of antiseptic mineral or vegetable oil instead of air for forcible lung compression reduced the risk of tuberculous empyema and the need for repeat procedure.
- **Phrenic nerve crush:** Paralysing the ipsilateral hemidiaphragm to the tuberculous foci reduced oxygenation. Success was seen in lower lobe granulomas when used in combination with pneumothorax techniques.
- **Plombage:** For patients unsuitable for external thoracoplasty compression or with bilateral disease, a combination of inert paraffin and bismuth was injected into the pleural cavity, forcibly compressing the adjacent lung. The use of inert Lucite (poly(methyl methacrylate)) balls was a later development but had characteristic appearances (Figure 97.2).

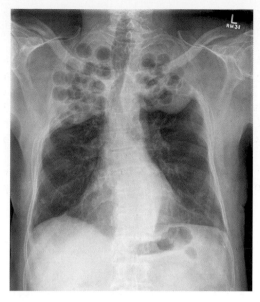

Figure 97.2 Appearance of Lucite balls on chest radiograph. Reproduced from Life in the Fast Lane medical blog, www.lifeinthefastlane.com, with permission.

 KEY POINTS

- Thoracoplasty for the treatment of *Mycobacterium tuberculosis* infection is still practised in developing countries.
- First to seventh ribs are often surgically removed with compression of the superior lateral chest wall.
- Before chemotherapy, 'collapse therapy' was deemed a 'ray of sunshine in the history of tuberculosis'.

References

1. Phillips, M.S., Kinnear, W.J.M. and Shneerson, J.M. (1987) Late sequelae of pulmonary tuberculosis treated by thoracoplasty. *Thorax* 42: 445–51.
2. Dewan, R.K., Singh, S., Kumar, A. and Meena, B.K. (1999) Thoracoplasty: an obsolete procedure? *Indian Journal of Chest Diseases and Allied Sciences* 41(2): 83–88.
3. Broenrigg, G.M. (1949) Thoracoplasty for pulmonary tuberculosis. *Canadian Medical Association Journal* 61: 601–602.
4. Singer, J.J. (1936) Collapse therapy in tuberculosis. *California and Western Medicine* 45(2): 120–25.

History

A 72-year-old woman is referred by her general practitioner (GP). She complains of sudden onset of back pain while playing with her grandchild 6 weeks ago and although her pain is now much better with analgesia, her symptoms have not resolved completely. She denies any history of direct trauma. Her pain is aching in character centred on her thoracic spine with stabbing exacerbations on certain movements, limiting her mobility. She does not complain of any numbness, tingling or pins and needles. She is able to walk and move all four limbs independently with no complaints of bowel or bladder disturbance. She has had no weight loss, change in bowel habit or any stigmata of infection.

Her past medical history includes bowel cancer 3 years ago treated with a right hemicolectomy. She has had no problems since.

Examination

She had a computed tomography (CT) scan performed 1 week ago as part of her continued surveillance. This did not report any evidence of local recurrence but did reveal an abnormality on bone review (Figure 98.1).

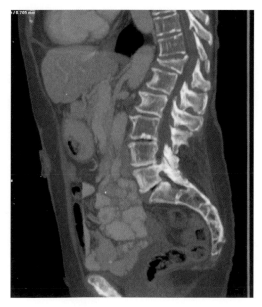

Figure 98.1 CT scan.

Questions

- What does this image demonstrate and what type of image is it?
- What is a bone scan?
- What is the likely cause of this patient's problems?

The image displayed in Figure 98.1 is a maximal intensity projection (MIP) of the lower thoracic, lumbar and sacral spine, reconstructed in the sagittal plane. MIPs are a type of post-processing technique regularly used in CT, and although MIP physics are out of the remit of this answer, they allow for both 2- and 3-dimensional reconstruction for improved diagnostic interpretation.

The image has been windowed to improve bony resolution. There has been collapse and loss of height of T12 in its anterior aspect with relative preservation of the vertebral body posteriorly in keeping with a wedge compression fracture. There is resultant kyphosis. Coronal imaging (Figure 98.2) confirms uniform loss of vertebral body height anteriorly, which is accentuated more on the right than the left.

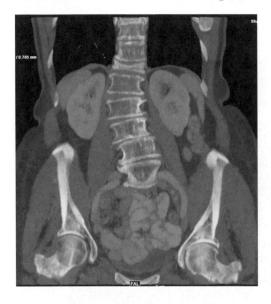

Figure 98.2 Coronal image.

There are many causes of vertebral body collapse, with the most common being trauma, malignancy and osteoporosis. Patients often complain of associated back pain and can have neurological symptoms if there is bony encroachment of the adjacent spinal canal with either cord or nerve compromise. The shape of the vertebral collapse can also be seen to change the normal curvature of the thoracic spine, and in elderly people suffering multilevel osteoporotic fractures, this can cause an overall loss of vertical height and a severe kyphoscoliosis.

It is important to establish a cause for the vertebral collapse, so that steps can be taken to prevent deterioration, multilevel involvement and a potential neurological deficit. Having excluded a history of trauma, the main differential lies between loss of vertebral bone integrity related to either malignancy or osteoporosis. Although it is impossible to say with certainty that a vertebral collapse on CT is due to osteoporosis rather than malignancy, other radiological studies can be employed to help distinguish between them. A bone scan can be very helpful and is discussed below, with a magnetic resonance imaging (MRI) scan often performed not only to diagnose any evidence of neurological compromise, but to define characteristic features of acute vertebral collapse that can infer one cause rather than the other. The infiltrative process of malignancy often causes diffuse loss of normal bone marrow signalling on T1 imaging and post-gadolinium; abnormal enhancement may be demonstrated with or without an associated epidural soft tissue mass. As some fatty marrow is maintained in osteoporosis, associated vertebral collapse often retains its concave posterior wall and is more likely solitary, as multilevel involvement is more in keeping with malignancy.

A bone scan (also referred to as 'bone scintigraphy') is a common type of nuclear medicine study that utilizes the normal physiological response to any bony insult, whether it be malignant, infective or osteoporotic. The radiotracer technetium-99m is chemically attached to methylene-diphosphate (MDP), and is preferentially taken up by osteoblasts when intravenously injected into the body and incorporated into the matrix of healing bone via hydroxyapatite deposition. Decay of this radioactive isotope is recorded on a gamma camera and generates a skeletal image of normal physiological uptake with 'hot-spots' of radioisotope accumulation at sites of bony injury. Interpretation of the distribution of tracer uptake can both imply an aetiology and also reveal other sites of abnormality that were previously clinically invisible.

In the bone scan of the same patient, there is a focal region of increased tracer uptake to the right of T12 and to the left of the lower lumbar vertebrae (Figure 98.3). Mild tracer uptake is also noted at the shoulders, knees, ankles and feet. The appearances are suggestive of vertebral degenerative collapse related to osteoporosis in keeping with the given CT images, however a solitary metastasis cannot be excluded. Tracer uptake in the joints is suggestive of further degenerative disease. Multiple 'hot-spots' suggest skeletal metastases have not been demonstrated.

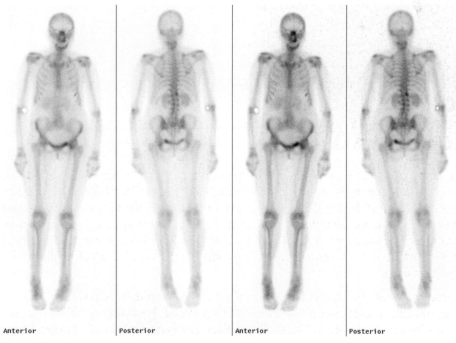

Anterior   Posterior   Anterior   Posterior

Figure 98.3 Bone scan.

 KEY POINTS

- CT scans have a high sensitivity at resolving bony pathology.
- If there is clinical suspicion of spinal cord involvement then an MRI study needs to be performed. MRI can help differentiate between osteoporosis and metastatic collapse.
- Bone scintigraphy can reveal sites of bony involvement that are clinically invisible.

History

A 78-year-old woman was transferred from the local nursing home complaining of abdominal pain and vomiting. She has been suffering from intermittent colicky abdominal pain for several years with no clear exacerbating or relieving factors. The pain comes on gradually, centred on the lower abdomen, and usually lasts a few hours before resolving spontaneously. It is often associated with nausea but never vomiting. She has been extensively investigated with computed tomography (CT) and a colonoscopy, but these were performed when the patient was asymptomatic and found no abnormality.

A typical episode started last night but the pain has failed to resolve by itself. She has not passed any faeces or flatus for 12 hours and complains of abdominal distension. She has a past medical history of hip replacements, diet-controlled diabetes and coronary artery disease. She has a long history of constipation and has been on laxative treatment for the last 20 years. She denies weight loss or recent change in bowel habit.

Examination

A plain abdominal radiograph was performed as part of the initial investigations (Figure 99.1).

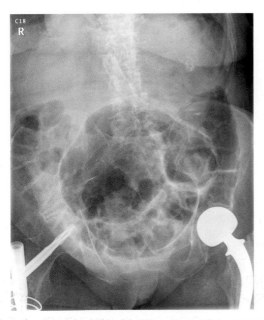

Figure 99.1 Abdominal radiograph.

Questions

- What does this radiograph demonstrate?
- What is the diagnosis and is there a differential for these appearances?
- Can this affect other parts of the body?

Figure 99.1 is a plain abdominal radiograph of an elderly patient with a background of degenerative bony change and bilateral hip replacements. There are dilated loops of large bowel extending from the caecum round to the sigmoid colon with maximal bowel diameter of 7 cm. The small bowel is decompressed and there is a paucity of gas within the rectum. Centrally, there is an isolated loop of grossly dilated large bowel that assumes an oval configuration centred on a linear density in the left lower quadrant. This is the characteristic 'coffee-bean' sign of sigmoid volvulus. There is no evidence of intra-abdominal free gas to suggest bowel perforation (Figure 99.2).

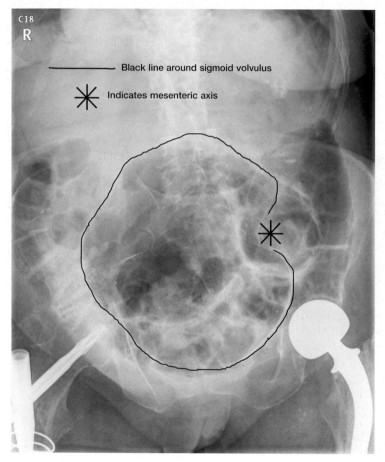

Figure 99.2 Abdominal radiograph indicating mesenteric axis and volvulus.

Volvulus is defined as twisting of the intestinal tract around a mesenteric axis. It is relatively rare but most commonly seen within the colon where it accounts for one in ten causes of large bowel obstruction. The mid- and hindgut is associated with a fold of fibro-fatty tissue called the mesentery, which provides mechanical support and carries nerves, blood vessels and lymphatics to the bowel. Anchored to the back of the abdominal wall, those loops of bowel that lie furthest from the mesenteric root are more mobile and can be susceptible to rotation. In the large bowel, the caecum and sigmoid colon are the commonest sites of involvement, with predisposing factors including an unusually long mesentery or chronic constipation.

Rotating around a mesenteric axis, the bowel twists and closes the lumen, causing bowel obstruction. This can resolve spontaneously in response to peristalsis, with patients complaining of intermittent resolving abdominal pain. Failure to untwist the bowel will cause bowel dilatation proximal to the obstruction with symptoms of pain, abdominal distension and vomiting. Patients may also have abdominal compartment syndrome because of the mass effect from the dilated bowel loop. Blood vessels supplying the involved segment of bowel are subject to strangulation, and this can lead to bowel ischaemia and infarction. Without definitive treatment, this carries a high mortality.

Differentiating between caecal and sigmoid volvulus can be difficult on plain radiograph:

- **Sigmoid** is commonly seen in the elderly with plain film findings of an isolated enlarged loop of large bowel centred on the left side with cranial extension towards the diaphragm. A midline fold that represents the twisted mesenteric axis can be seen, causing the characteristic 'coffee-bean' appearance (arrow). There is often associated transverse and ascending colon dilatation, with normal small bowel calibre if the ileo-caecal valve is competent.
- **Caecal** is a disease of the young (averaging 30 years) with the dilated caecum rotating anteriorly and lying in the left upper quadrant. This is associated with small bowel dilatation and puts the patient at increased risk of bowel perforation.

Other types of volvulus include the following:

- **Gastric:** Rotation of the stomach around the supportive gastrohepatic (lesser curve) or gastrocolic (greater curve) mesenteries can cause sudden onset severe abdominal pain and vomiting. It is considered a surgical emergency carrying up to 80 per cent mortality if treatment is not initiated quickly. There are two types: organoaxial (rotating in a vertical axis, imaging reveals the characteristic appearances of a 'mirror-image' stomach with the greater curve within the right upper quadrant) and mesenteroaxial (rotating along a horizontal axis, the stomach appears to be upside down with the pylorus seen at the expected gastro-oesophageal junction).
- **Midgut volvulus** (described in Case 88): This is associated with congenital malrotation. Seen primarily in infants, the midgut rotates around the superior mesenteric artery (SMA) axis, causing bowel obstruction and the characteristic 'double-bubble' sign on plain radiograph.

 KEY POINTS

- Volvulus occurs when a loop of bowel twists around a mesenteric axis.
- Look for the characteristic 'coffee-bean' sign to help differentiate between a sigmoid and caecal volvulus.
- Midgut volvulus is associated with congenital malrotation of the bowel.

History
A 27-year-old woman attends the accident and emergency department one morning unable to weight-bear on her right ankle. She had been out two nights before and consumed a large quantity of alcohol. She remembers falling, twisting her right ankle and subsequently being unable to walk well. This had been painful over the course of the next day and had kept her awake the previous night. She attended to check it was just a 'sprain'.

Examination
She is unable to weight-bear on the right. Upon examination, the right ankle was swollen, with reduced range of motion and there was bony tenderness upon bony palpation of the lateral malleolus (distal fibula). She was neurovascularly intact distally, with foot pulses and normal power/sensation in the foot. Radiographs were requested in the accident and emergency department (Figure 100.1).

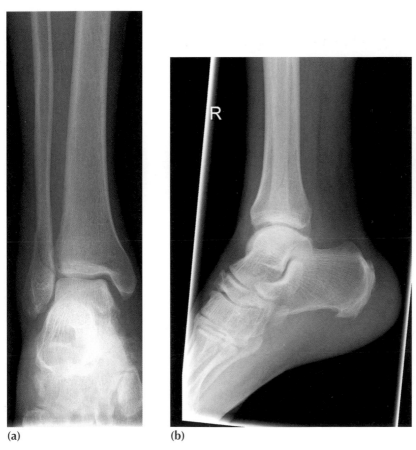

(a)　　　　　**(b)**

Figure 100.1 (a) Anterior–posterior (AP) and (b) lateral ankle radiographs.

Question
- What do the ankle radiographs demonstrate?

The radiographs (Figure 100.1a,b) demonstrate an undisplaced spiral fracture of the distal fibula (lateral malleolus) demonstrated with arrows on Figure 100.2.

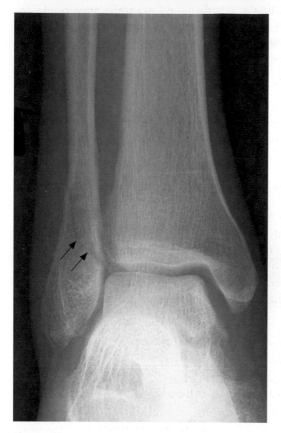

Figure 100.2

Ankle fractures are usually the result of low-energy twisting/torsion forces and present with swelling, deformity and inability to bear weight. Non-displaced ankle fractures may occasionally exhibit minimal swelling and no deformity.

Ankle fractures are one of the most common fractures treated by accident and emergency departments and comprise a range of different injury patterns, varying in severity. Isolated malleolar fractures make up approximately two-thirds of ankle fractures, with bimalleolar fractures occurring in a quarter, and trimalleolar fractures occurring in the remaining 7 per cent of cases. Open fractures occur in approximately 2 per cent of cases.

The ankle is often thought of as a simple hinge joint, although biomechanically the axis of rotation is constantly changing as the ankle allows variable degrees of rotation and translation in the coronal and axial planes as well as the sagittal plane.

The ankle joint is formed by contributions from the tibia, fibula and talus. When the foot is dorsiflexed, the widened anterior portion of the talus fits securely within the medial and lateral malleoli and the talocrural joint acts as a true mortise with the bony structures providing the majority of the stability. When the ankle moves into plantar flexion, the narrower portion of the talar dome articulates between the medial and lateral malleoli, where the talus does not fit as tightly (and the majority of the joint stability is conferred by surrounding ligaments).

A number of methods of classification exist for ankle fractures, however it is most important to simply describe the fracture, in particular whether the fracture is open or closed, the condition of the soft tissue (including swelling or blisters) and the bony structures involved (in particular, is it unimalleolar, bimalleolar or trimalleolar?). Further points may include the fracture pattern, amount of comminution and the status of the syndesmosis.

More systematized methods include the commonly used Lauge–Hansen Classification and Weber Classification:

- Lauge–Hansen Classification: This is based on the fracture pattern. Each configuration is defined by two factors: the position of the foot (pronation or supination) and the force applied to the ankle (adduction, external rotation or abduction). In addition each configuration has a number of stages describing sequential injuries as the force was applied, the most common mechanism being the supination–external rotation pattern.
- Weber Classification: This is a simple system for classification of lateral malleolar fractures relating to the level of the ankle joint and determining treatment. Fractures are divided into three categories based on the level of the fibula fracture in relation to the joint line (syndesmosis). Weber A fractures occur distal to the joint line, while Weber B fractures involve the syndesmosis and Weber C fractures are confined above the joint line. The fracture in this example would be an undisplaced Weber B fracture.

 KEY POINTS

- Isolated malleolar fractures make up approximately two-thirds of ankle fractures.
- These injuries may only be seen clearly on one view of the ankle, therefore two views are required in all cases of ankle trauma.

INDEX

Note: Reference are the form of case number with page numbers in brackets. There are main entries for all imaging modalities excluding 'radiograph' which occurs too frequently for indexing. There are though entries for the less-commonly used terms involving X-rays such as 'chest radiograph', 'contrast studies', 'fluoroscopy' and 'X-ray physics'.